OXFORD MEDICAL PUBLICATIONS

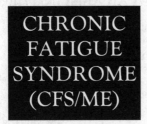

CHRONIC
FATIGUE
SYNDROME
(CFS/ME)

the**facts**

D1037587

the**facts**
ALSO AVAILABLE IN THE SERIES

ALCOHOLISM: THE FACTS
(third edition) Donald W. Goodwin

AUTISM: THE FACTS
Simon Baron-Cohen and
Patrick Bolton

BACK AND NECK PAIN:
THE FACTS
Loïc Burn

CANCER: THE FACTS
(second edition) Michael Whitehouse
and Maurice Slevin

CHILDHOOD LEUKAEMIA:
THE FACTS
(second edition) John S. Lilleyman

CHRONIC FATIGUE SYNDROME
(CFS/ME): THE FACTS
Frankie Campling and Michael Sharpe

CYSTIC FIBROSIS: THE FACTS
(third edition) Ann Harris and
Maurice Super

DOWN SYNDROME: THE FACTS
(second edition) Mark Selikowitz

DYSLEXIA AND OTHER
LEARNING DIFFICULTIES:
THE FACTS
(second edition) Mark Selikowitz

EATING DISORDERS:
THE FACTS
(fourth edition) Suzanne Abraham and
Derek Llewellyn-Jones

ECZEMA IN CHILDHOOD:
THE FACTS
David J. Atherton

EPILEPSY: THE FACTS
(second edition) Anthony Hopkins
and Richard Appleton

HEAD INJURY: THE FACTS
(second edition) Dorothy Gronwall,
Philip Wrightson, and Peter Waddell

HUNTINGTON'S DISEASE:
THE FACTS
Oliver Quarrell

KIDNEY FAILURE: THE FACTS
Stewart Cameron

LUPUS: THE FACTS
Graham Hughes

MISCARRIAGE: THE FACTS
(second edition) Gillian C.L. Lachelin

MUSCULAR DYSTROPHY:
THE FACTS
(second edition) Alan E.H. Emery

OBSESSIVE-COMPULSIVE
DISORDER: THE FACTS
(second edition) Padmal de Silva and
Stanley Rachman

PANIC DISORDER: THE FACTS
Stanley Rachman and Padmal de Silva

SCHIZOPHRENIA: THE FACTS
(second edition) Ming T. Tsuang and
Stephen V. Faraone

THYROID DISEASE: THE FACTS
(third edition) R.I.S. Bayliss and
W.M.G. Tunbridge

TOURETTE SYNDROME:
THE FACTS
(second edition) Mary Robertson and
Simon Baron-Cohen

ALSO FROM OXFORD
UNIVERSITY PRESS

FORBIDDEN DRUGS
UNDERSTANDING DRUGS AND
WHY PEOPLE TAKE THEM
(second edition) Philip Robson

A BLOKE'S DIAGNOSE IT
YOURSELF GUIDE TO HEALTH
Keith Hopcroft and Alistair Moulds

CHRONIC FATIGUE SYNDROME (CFS/ME)

the**facts**

Frankie Campling
a person with CFS/ME
and
Michael Sharpe
*Senior Lecturer and Honorary Consultant
in Psychological Medicine
The University of Edinburgh
Scotland, UK*

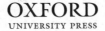

OXFORD
UNIVERSITY PRESS

OXFORD
UNIVERSITY PRESS

Great Clarendon Street, Oxford OX2 6DP

Oxford University Press is a department of the University of Oxford
and furthers the University's aim of excellence in research, scholarship,
and education by publishing worldwide in

Oxford New York

Athens Auckland Bangkok Bogota Buenos Aires Calcutta
Cape Town Chennai Dar es Salaam Delhi Florence Hong Kong Istanbul
Karachi Kuala Lumpur Madrid Melbourne Mexico City Mumbai
Nairobi Paris São Paulo Singapore Taipei Tokyo Toronto Warsaw

and associated companies in Berlin Ibadan

Oxford is a trade mark of Oxford University Press

Published in the United States
by Oxford University Press Inc., New York

© Frankie Campling and Michael Sharpe, 2000

A catalogue record for this title is available from the British Library

Library of Congress Cataloging in Publication Data
(Data available)
1 3 5 7 9 10 8 6 4 2

ISBN 0 19 263049 0

Typeset by Downdell, Oxford
Printed in Great Britain by
Biddles Ltd., Guildford & King's Lynn

the**facts**

CONTENTS

Section 1

Chronic fatigue syndrome: its nature, diagnosis, and treatment

Section 2

The idea of self-help

Contents

Section 3
Special issues

Appendices

Index

Introduction

This book is addressed primarily to people suffering from chronic fatigue syndrome (CFS/ME), their carers, families, and friends. We also hope that other people who want to understand more about this illness may read it. We wish to stress, right from the outset, that we understand that people suffering from CFS/ME have a genuine, distressing, and debilitating illness. We also believe that there is much that can be done to help.

Both authors have wide experience of the illness going back more than ten years—Frankie Campling as a person with CFS/ME who does telephone support work for others like herself and Michael Sharpe as a clinician and researcher who has run specialist clinical services for CFS/ME and has published widely on the illness. Our combined experience enables us to see the illness from the perspectives of both medical science and sufferers. We hope that this collaboration of doctor and patient will offer our readers a unique perspective on CFS/ME, on what doctors can do to help, and especially on what sufferers can do to help themselves.

Our main aims in writing this book were:

- to explain what is meant by CFS/ME and how it is diagnosed;
- to provide research-based information on possible causes and treatments;

- to help our readers to evaluate new findings and claims about CFS/ME;
- to help patients and carers make informed decisions about treatment;
- to offer practical guidance on what patients can do to help themselves.

We know that many people with CFS/ME suffer greatly because those around them do not believe that they are ill, or even suggest that the illness is imaginary or 'all in the mind'. This is such an important subject that we discuss it in detail, suggesting why this disbelief occurs, reviewing evidence that indicates that CFS/ME is a 'real' illness, and suggesting ways of communicating with family, friends, and doctors that will minimize this most distressing problem.

Having said that, you may be surprised to find that we spend a good deal of time discussing behavioural and psychological strategies for the management of CFS/ME. This is because both the available research evidence and our own experience show that these are the most helpful treatments. Drug therapy has a role but the evidence for its effectiveness is less good. This does *not* mean that we believe that CFS/ME is a psychological illness. It is just that, as with all illnesses, the way a sufferer copes will influence both their quality of life and the outcome of the illness. And the fact that we do not yet fully understand the causes of CFS/ME does not mean that we are unable to work out how best to manage it.

We should stress that though we can offer you a 'map' of scientific information about CFS/ME and its treatment, you as a patient are the expert on the 'territory' of your own illness. We can offer you advice about management strategies that other patients have found helpful, but you are the one to choose whether or not to try them. All we ask is that you should approach what we write with an open mind.

We very much hope that you will want to try out the techniques we suggest. We believe that you will find, as others have, that they will improve your situation and that even if they do not produce a cure, they will give you a sense of greater control over the illness and optimism about the future.

One of the most important of the management strategies we discuss is that of pacing yourself carefully, always stopping before you get too tired. We suggest that you read this book in a similar way. Take it slowly. Do not try to read it all in one sitting. You will probably get more out of it if you read a chapter or two and then stop for a rest. We have tried to keep our language simple. However, we are aware that you may still come across unfamiliar medical words and so have included a glossary of such words at the back of the book.

In conclusion, we hope that you will find this book helpful and that it will improve your understanding of CFS/ME. We also hope that it will give you ideas about what *you* can do to improve both your state of health and your quality of life.

Acknowledgements

We are very grateful to those people, both clinicians and patients, who read the manuscript and gave us such valuable comments and suggestions. These include Hilary Briars, Dr John Campling, Dr Zoe Dunhill, Dr Birgitta Evengard, Dr William Hamilton, Katherine Kephalas, Dr Ivana Klimes, Dr Andrew Lloyd, Dr Duncan Manders, Dr Peter White, and Dr David Wilks, though many others have given us really helpful assistance.

We thank James Campling and Elizabeth Sharpe for the support and encouragement they gave us while we were writing this book (and for their toleration of the process).

Most of all, though, we want to thank all the people with CFS/ME whom we have worked with over the last ten or more years. They have taught us so much about what suffering from CFS/ME is like and what they have found helpful. This book is dedicated to them.

Section 1
Chronic fatigue syndrome
(CFS/ME): its nature,
diagnosis, and treatment

1

Our aims in this section

The questions that get asked

If you or someone you know has been diagnosed as having chronic fatigue syndrome (or even if that is just what is suspected) you are likely to have a lot of questions you want answered. During the ten years and more that we have been working with those suffering from CFS/ME we have become familiar with the questions that get asked most frequently. These are:

- Is it a real illness?
- What should it be called?
- Why is it called that?
- What are the symptoms?
- Who gets it?
- What happens to them?
- How is it diagnosed?
- What is the cause?
- What is the best treatment?

Discussion about chronic fatigue syndrome often begins with such questions as *Does it really exist?* or *Is it a 'real' illness or is it 'all in the mind'?* These questions are based on a lack of understanding. They can be hurtful and unhelpful to patients suffering from the illness. In this section of the book we will review the known facts about chronic fatigue syndrome with the hope of overcoming such misunderstandings. We will also give some answers to the other questions.

How should we judge 'facts'?

The title of this book is 'Chronic fatigue syndrome (CFS/ME): the facts' because it is one in a series *The facts* published by Oxford University Press. You may already be aware that CFS/ME is an illness for which facts seem to be few whilst theories abound. We have tried to marshal for you what facts there are and have also attempted to offer the best information and advice on aspects of CFS/ME for which there are no undisputed facts. We have done this because we believe that moving forward with scepticism is preferable to being paralysed by uncertainty. In the chapters that follow we have tried to indicate which statements are facts, which are informed opinions, and which are merely ideas and anecdotes by pointing out the quality of evidence supporting them. We have distinguished three different types of evidence:

1. *Sound scientific research.* This is the level of evidence required by what has become known as 'evidence-based medicine'. When such evidence is available we have highlighted it. These are facts.

2. *Clinical experience.* This is where there is some research evidence that has been replicated and/or where there is a degree of consensus amongst health professionals working with patients who have CFS/ME. This is informed opinion.

3. *Anecdotal evidence.* This is the weakest evidence. It covers the area of disputed or unreplicated scientific reports and 'we have heard from some people that they have found such-and-such helpful'. These are merely ideas and anecdotes.

You should bear in mind the level of evidence for each statement when reading what we have to say here and do the same for what you read elsewhere. We would encourage you to be suitably sceptical where the evidence is weak.

In Appendix 4 we have included further reading and suggestions about how to evaluate information about CFS/ME in a critical way as you encounter it. You might wish to practise these suggestions by applying them to this book!

2

What shall we call it?

What's in a name?

Various names are used for this illness, which can be very confusing. What are the different names, and where do they come from? Do they all mean the same thing? What name should we use? Well, to start with the first question (and ignoring silly labels like 'yuppie flu'), the names used for this condition can be:

Chronic fatigue syndrome (CFS)

Chronic fatigue syndrome (CFS) is now the name most generally used by doctors and the one they mostly prefer. In medical language 'chronic' means that an illness has been present for a long time, usually more than six months. 'Chronic' is distinguished from 'acute' which means an illness of rapid and severe onset but often short duration. A syndrome is an illness or condition that is diagnosed on the basis of a combination of symptoms and/or signs (as opposed to abnormalities in tests). In CFS the symptom shared by all sufferers is severe fatigue. Other symptoms commonly present are muscle aches, poor concentration, and feeling unwell after exertion. (We will look at other symptoms in Chapter 3.)

Myalgic encephalomyelitis (ME)

This was a name given to an acute, medically unexplained illness that occurred in the 1950s among the staff of the Royal Free Hospital, London. Many doctors do not agree with applying this name to patients with chronic fatigue symptoms for two reasons. The first is that many of the symptoms of the Royal Free outbreak were different from those experienced by CFS patients today. The second is that this name is potentially misleading as although many patients do have myalgia (this simply means muscle pain), there is no good evidence that they have encephalomyelitis (inflammation of the brain and spinal cord). However, ME is a name commonly used by patients, the general public, the media, and some doctors.

Chronic fatigue and immune dysfunction syndrome (CFIDS)

Patients and some doctors in the USA use this name. It highlights not only the fatigue but also immune changes. Relatively small changes can be found in the functioning of the immune system in some patients (as they can in many illnesses). However, it is still not clear how important these are in causing the symptoms. Furthermore, the apparent similarity with the term AIDS (acquired immune deficiency syndrome), in which there is an important and severe disturbance of immune functioning, is potentially misleading (and unnecessarily worrying).

Post-viral fatigue syndrome (PVFS)

This label is sometimes used by doctors in cases which appear to have started with a viral illness. 'Post-viral' simply means after a virus. It does not necessarily mean that a virus is causing the continuing condition. As viral infections are very common it can be difficult to be certain whether any one viral infection was the cause or not. The term does not really mean anything different from CFS.

Neurasthenia

This name was used in the late-1800s to describe a condition that was probably much the same as CFS. The term literally means 'weak nerves'. Later on, this diagnosis fell out of favour—although doctors still occasionally use it.

Names of epidemics

Other names sometimes used refer to places where a number of patients became ill with something simi-lar—Los Angeles and Akureyri are examples. The relationship of these apparent epidemics to the more common cases is unclear. These names are therefore best avoided for routine use.

Why do most doctors call it chronic fatigue syndrome?

The term 'chronic fatigue syndrome' was officially coined in the late-1980s. Prior to that time people suffering from severe and chronic fatigue that could not be medically explained were given a variety of diagnoses. One common diagnosis was infection with Epstein–Barr virus (EBV), the virus that causes glandular fever. Other infections blamed included chronic Brucellosis (a rare infection transmitted from cows).

By the 1980s, however, it was becoming clear to researchers that the accumulating scientific evidence did not support the idea that these infections were the cause of the chronic fatigue in most cases. In 1988 a group of physicians met at the Centers for Disease Control (CDC) in Atlanta, USA, to discuss this matter. They chose the name chronic fatigue syndrome (CFS). This name was preferred because it simply described the illness (although emphasizing one symptom) and did not make any assumptions about the cause, which they agreed was unknown. Researchers in the UK and Australia also agreed independently to use this name. These various groups of medical researchers hoped that admitting their ignorance about the cause would stimulate research and that an agreed name would make it easier for them to communicate with each other about their findings.

What is wrong with the name 'chronic fatigue syndrome'?

Many patients are unhappy about their illness being called chronic fatigue syndrome. There are two main reasons for this. Patients say that the emphasis on fatigue has had the effect of trivializing their suffering and disability—encouraging comments such as 'well we all get tired you know'. They also say that highlighting the one symptom of fatigue ignores their other symptoms (which are often more distressing to them).

Not surprisingly, therefore, there have been campaigns to have the name changed. Some of these have favoured an eponym—using the name of someone well known who has studied the illness (such as Melvin Ramsay) or someone who apparently suffered from it (such as Florence Nightingale). Others have favoured a name that sounds more like a medical disease than CFS (such as myalgic encephalopathy—a different version of ME).

Changing the name would not be easy. The term CFS is established in medical journals and textbooks (and on most scientific databases), so doctors and researchers would have to cooperate in changing it. It seems likely that any change in name will have to await research findings that offer a new understanding of the cause of the illness or illnesses currently referred to as CFS.

So do these names all refer to the same illness?

The names in common usage today probably do all refer to much the same collection of symptoms, though they differ in their historical origins and in what they imply about the nature of the illness. However, it seems increasingly likely that patients with chronic fatigue syndrome do not all have exactly the same condition even though they may experience somewhat similar symptoms. This is what doctors mean when they talk of a 'heterogeneous' condition. In time, different subgroups may be identified.

Some people believe that there is a subgroup of patients with CFS who have a particularly severe illness (which they would prefer to be called ME), which should be researched and treated differently than CFS. This suggestion may be correct, but it has not yet been proved.

The name we are using

Chronic fatigue syndrome (CFS) is the current medically preferred name for the illness and so we will use it. However, the term ME is also used very often to refer to the same illness (particularly by patients), so we have decided to use the combined term 'CFS/ME' in this book.

There are a number of different names that have been or are still being used to label this illness. In general, they refer to similar, if not identical, conditions and so are largely interchangeable. In due course research may allow the illness to be split into different subtypes. At present, chronic fatigue syndrome (CFS) is the name most favoured by doctors. Some patients prefer ME. In this book we will use the combined term CFS/ME.

3
What is chronic fatigue syndrome (CFS/ME)?

What is fatigue?

As 'fatigue' forms part of the medical name, it seems sensible to talk about that first. People often mean different things when they talk about fatigue. They may mean a feeling of sleepiness, a reluctance to start a task, an inability to keep going at a task, or feeling terrible after exertion. Fatigue may also refer to the normal weariness experienced after having worked hard. These varied meanings are a source of confusion. It is important when talking about fatigue to specify what sort of fatigue we mean. Certainly the fatigue experienced by people with CFS/ME is very different from 'everyday' tiredness.

When is fatigue an illness?

Fatigue is very common. Surveys have shown that almost a quarter of the population, if asked, will say that fatigue has been a problem for them over the last month. Fatigue of some degree is normal and often related to periods of stress, overwork, depression, or loss of sleep. People usually consult a doctor about fatigue when it is both persistent and sufficiently severe to interfere with daily activities. This is when fatigue becomes a major problem for patients and clinically significant to doctors. It may then be considered as an illness.

Types of fatiguing illness

Persistent severe fatigue can be caused by many diseases. The type of fatigue may give a clue to the nature of the disease. For example, fatigue that is described as an overwhelming need to fall asleep points to a sleep problem. Fatigue that feels like a loss of motivation, interest, and enjoyment (sometimes called anhedonia) suggests depression. The typical fatigue of CFS/ME is described as a feeling of exhaustion, weariness, and debility that makes it difficult to start or persist in a physical or mental task and that is made worse by the effort of attempting it. People with CFS/ME usually say that their fatigue is very different from the tiredness they experienced before they were ill and describe it as not just feeling exhausted but really ill. Persistent, severe fatigue of this type that restricts normal activity and is not explained by another condition may lead to a diagnosis of CFS/ME.

A research definition of CFS/ME

When the name CFS was coined in 1988 by the Centers

for Disease Control (CDC) in Atlanta, USA, it was linked to a detailed definition of the illness. This first definition was made so that the label could be used in the same way by all researchers. However, because the definition proposed proved difficult to use in practice, it was later altered.

In 1991 a group of British clinicians and researchers met in Oxford, UK, and agreed on what are now known as the 'Oxford criteria' for CFS (criteria mean standards by which something is judged). In 1994 the CDC decided to revise its own case definition based on the consensus of researchers from several countries. It was similar to the one agreed in Oxford. The main changes from the original definition were to allow patients who also suffered from depression and anxiety to be described as having chronic fatigue syndrome and to reduce the number of symptoms required other than fatigue. (In case you are interested, we have included the exact definitions of both the Oxford and the 1994 International CDC criteria as Appendix 3.)

Today the 1991 Oxford and the 1994 International CDC definitions are the currently accepted definitions for CFS. However, there is nothing absolute about these criteria. They were constructed by committees (do you know the joke that a camel is a horse designed by a committee?) and were intended to provide standard definitions for *research* studies, not for clinical practice where diagnoses may be made and used more pragmatically. They will be reviewed and it is likely that at some point in the future, when our understanding of the processes that give rise to the symptoms of CFS is better, they will be superseded. For the moment they are the best we have.

The main parts of the current definitions are:

- the symptom of severe fatigue
- other specified symptoms
- a reduced level of activity
- an illness lasting at least six months
- no better medical explanation for the fatigue.

An extended period with the symptoms was specified in order to separate CFS from the brief fatigue states that can occur after almost any illness (although the precise figure of six months is arbitrary).

What other symptoms?

The symptoms listed in the International CDC definition of CFS/ME are:

- malaise (feeling ill) after exertion
- difficulties with memory and concentration
- sore throat
- tender lymph nodes ('glands' in the neck, armpit, and groin)
- myalgia (muscle pain)
- arthralgia (joint pain)
- headaches
- disturbed and unrefreshing sleep.

As well as these symptoms, people with CFS/ME often experience others. These can include:

- abdominal and digestive problems
- chest pains

- nausea (feeling sick)
- feeling inappropriately hot or cold
- night sweats
- looking pale when tired
- feeling dizzy or light-headed
- problems with balance
- worsening of symptoms before a period
- hearing problems such as hyperacusis (painful sensitivity to noises)
- eye problems such as pain round the eyes, difficulty focusing, and sensitivity to bright lights.

Some of these symptoms can be frightening. You may fear that they indicate a life-threatening disease. If you have moments like this, do discuss your fears with your doctor. In Chapter 4 we will tell you about the routine medical tests you are likely to have had and what conditions they will have ruled out.

Is CFS/ME real?

One of the most difficult issues for both patients and doctors when a diagnosis of CFS/ME is made is how to understand it. What sort of illness is it that does not show up on any tests? Some people (and that includes some doctors) believe inaccurately that normal test results mean that there is really nothing wrong. This may lead to patients feeling that their complaints have been ignored, that they have been accused of making them up, or that their problem is 'purely mental' or 'all in the mind'. To make matters worse, many people tend to regard those illnesses thought of as 'mental' as an indication that a person is weak, at fault, or even malingering.

These misconceptions can be very upsetting, but they *are* misconceptions. They result from two errors. The first error is the belief that standard *medical* tests can detect all disturbances in bodily functioning. They cannot, but, as they say, 'absence of evidence does not mean evidence of absence'. However, in patients with CFS/ME and other related 'unexplained' illnesses, *research* tests can frequently detect disturbances in the functioning of the body and especially some in the nervous system.

The second error is the belief that people can be regarded as being made of two separate parts—a 'mind' and a 'body'. This is an outmoded 'dualistic' way of thinking about illness. A more modern view is that mind and body are not separate but rather are two sides of the same coin. For instance, states of mind have parallel states of brain.

We suggest that dividing illness into categories of *either* mental/psychiatric *or* physical/medical categories is a serious and potentially harmful mistake. Rather, there are physical, psychological, and social aspects of all illnesses—including CFS/ME.

How common is CFS/ME?

You may remember that earlier we mentioned surveys in which it was found that almost a quarter of the population complain of a problem with fatigue. CFS/ME is, of course, a good deal less common than that. Available studies suggest that it is present in between

2 in every thousand (0.2%) to 20 in every thousand (2.0%) of the population.

What sorts of people get CFS/ME?

CFS/ME can occur at any age and can affect people with all sorts of occupations or income level. Specialized hospital clinics do tend to have a higher proportion of well-educated, professional patients but that may be due to those people's greater ability to get themselves referred to such clinics. CFS/ME does seem to occur more often in women than in men, though it is not clear why this should be so.

What is the outcome (or 'prognosis') of CFS/ME?

The majority of people with CFS/ME improve. The illness is usually at its worst in the first few months and tends to improve thereafter. It is important to stress that for most people this illness does not lead to long-term severe disability. However, recovery can be a slow process and often takes the form of a frustrating 'up and down' pattern of improvements and setbacks.

Some people make a complete recovery, while others feel improved but would not regard themselves as having returned to full health. Unfortunately, a minority of people do remain chronically ill for reasons that are not well understood. These differing outcomes may reflect different types of CFS/ME. They probably also reflect the different ways in which patients respond to and cope with the illness. By managing your illness as well as possible you will give yourself the best chance of improvement and recovery. We discuss what 'good management' means in the second section of this book.

Fatigue is very common in the general population. Severe chronic disabling fatigue is much less common. It can be a symptom of a number of illnesses, especially stress and depression. People who are suffering from severe fatigue may get a diagnosis of CFS/ME if they have:

1. severe fatigue that limits their ability to do things;

2. a number of other symptoms;

3. no other known medical condition that could produce similar symptoms.

CFS/ME can affect anyone, although it is more common in women. Most people improve, although the degree of recovery varies. You can give yourself the best chance of improvement by following the advice included in Section 2 of this book.

4

How a diagnosis of CFS/ ME is made

A diagnosis of CFS/ME is made on the basis of the patient's symptoms and history. There are no findings on examination (clinical signs) in CFS/ME and so far no definitive medical test that can positively identify this condition. The physical examination and the laboratory investigations or 'tests' are important to exclude other conditions that could be causing the symptoms.

Ruling out other conditions

To do this, the doctor assessing you will listen to your history, examine you, and arrange any necessary tests. In this way he or she will rule out other diseases. This is important. If you were found to have another disease that is readily treatable or even life-threatening (which CFS/ME is not) you would receive different treatment.

The list of conditions that can cause the symptoms similar to those of CFS/ME is a long one. However, your doctor will be unlikely to need to ask questions about or do tests for *all* of these conditions. This would be time-consuming, potentially hazardous to you, and very expensive. Instead, he or she will only test for those conditions that are either very common or that your history (and physical examination) suggests as a possible explanation for the symptoms in your case. The most important way of finding out what is wrong is by asking the patient about their illness—which is called 'taking a history'.

Further history

The doctor may want to ask you about other symptoms in order to obtain more information to help to make a diagnosis. As depression and anxiety are among the most common causes of fatigue, your doctor is also likely to consider whether these could be a factor in your case and to ask about other symptoms that could suggest these (see Chapters 5 and 22). Having depression or anxiety does not mean that you cannot also have CFS/ME—but it makes sense to diagnose and treat these conditions if present and then see what symptoms are left. Your doctor will also ask about other symptoms that might suggest other diseases.

Physical examination

Having taken a history the doctor will usually conduct a physical examination. Depending on what he or she has learned from the history this may be a very limited one or may be a full examination requiring that you undress.

Laboratory tests

Some very common illnesses should probably be tested for in everyone who has chronic fatigue. These are anaemia, evidence of inflammation or infection, disturbance of blood chemistry due to liver, kidney, or hormonal dysfunction, and a low level of thyroid hormone and diabetes mellitus. The tests for these are:

Test	What it rules out
Full blood count	Anaemia
	Infection
ESR (erythrocyte sedimentation rate)	Infection or inflammation
CRP (C reactive protein)	Infection or inflammation
Urea and electrolytes	Kidney problems. Problems with the level of sodium and potassium in the blood
Liver function tests	Problems with the liver
T3/T4/TSH	Problems with the thyroid gland
Urine/blood glucose	Diabetes mellitus

Other conditions which can cause fatigue

There are other less common conditions that may need to be excluded in a few people. The list is long. In fact, most known diseases can cause fatigue. However, these less common diseases are only rarely found in people with the typical symptoms of CFS/ME. Most of these diseases are treatable. We cannot provide a complete list but have given some examples of medical conditions that cause fatigue and might be considered by your doctor:

- If you have a lot of joint and muscle pain, your doctor may do tests for a range of rheumatic diseases. Rarer 'autoimmune' diseases (where the body's own immune system causes damage to bodily organs) often cause joint pain and fatigue. Your doctor will usually be alerted to this possibility by findings on examination or from standard blood tests.

- Some gastrointestinal diseases may lead to fatigue. They usually cause diarrhoea and weight loss. If you have predominant gastric symptoms, your doctor may arrange for tests to exclude such conditions. One such condition is coeliac disease, which is caused by inflammation of the small intestine due to a reaction to the gluten in certain cereals (wheat, barley, and rye). The treatment is a gluten-free diet and is usually completely effective.

- Neurological diseases can present with fatigue. Multiple sclerosis usually causes loss of power or sensation in part of the body and can also cause fatigue. Myasthenia gravis is a rare condition in which there is a problem between muscles and the nerves that make them work. It causes weakness. Both have treatments.

- Hormonal conditions can lead to fatigue. A routine test of urine/blood glucose for diabetes may be appropriate, as may a blood test for an underactive thyroid gland. An endocrine condition called Addison's disease (due to inadequate functioning of the adrenal gland) also causes fatigue but is very rare. Giving the missing hormone can treat all these conditions.

- Infections can certainly cause fatigue. Examples include viral hepatitis, Lyme disease, glandular fever (Epstein–Barr virus), and Q fever. These infections can trigger fatigue. Less commonly they can persist. They are relatively uncommon causes of chronic fatigue.

• Severe sleep problems, such as a condition called sleep apnoea syndrome, can cause daytime fatigue, mainly sleepiness. Sleep apnoea is when a person stops breathing briefly many times during the night, often in association with loud snoring. It is diagnosed by having sleep and breathing measured overnight in a sleep laboratory. It can be treated.

Expensive and sophisticated tests

If your doctor suspects that you might be suffering from another condition, further specialist tests might be done. For example, if there is something that suggests that you could have a problem with the nerves in your arms or legs, electrical equipment may be used to test the nerves (this is called neurophysiological testing). If a disease is suspected which would have a visible effect on the brain, a CT (computerized tomography) or an MRI (magnetic resonance imaging) scan might be done to obtain a picture of the brain. These scans are *not* a test for CFS/ME, as the results in patients with the illness are typically normal. They do provide a means of excluding other brain diseases. MRI scans are particularly sensitive at detecting multiple sclerosis (MS).

A reassuring note

Research shows that once patients who have the symptoms of CFS/ME have been seen and assessed by a doctor, the chance that other possible causes have been missed is small. Once patients have been seen by several doctors, that chance becomes even smaller. However, it is not possible to exclude all diseases conclusively. If your symptoms change it may be wise to tell your doctor and not to assume automatically that every new symptom is due to CFS/ME. On the other hand, it really is unhelpful to focus too much on your symptoms. This simply holds you back from recovery and gets in the way of enjoying life.

After the tests

When your doctor has ruled out all the other things that might be causing the symptoms, he or she can say that it is probably CFS/ME. If you had a viral infection at the beginning of your illness your doctor may call it post-viral fatigue syndrome (PVFS).

You may find it helpful to ask your doctor what tests have been performed and what has been ruled out. At least then you will know what you do *not* have. Do remember that if your doctor says, 'all the tests are normal', he or she is *not* saying that you are not feeling ill. It just means that you do not have any of the medical conditions that these tests show up. The lack of a definitive medical test for CFS/ME does not mean that the illness does not exist, or that it is 'all in your mind'.

Some doctors are reluctant to give patients a diagnosis of CFS/ME because they believe that not enough is known about it and that it is not a proper or helpful diagnosis. This is understandable from the doctor's point of view, but it often leaves patients in a difficult position. It is hard for anyone to make sense of their illness or to deal with it in the best way without a diagnosis. If your doctor prefers not to make a diagnosis it may be helpful to explain this to him or her.

A diagnosis of CFS/ME is made by excluding other diseases that might cause severe chronic fatigue and associated symptoms. Most common conditions causing similar symptoms can be ruled out by asking you questions, examining you, and conducting simple blood or urine tests. Your doctor may test for other rarer conditions if there is something in your history, symptoms, or examination that suggests this as a possibility. Although there is no definitive medical test for CFS/ME, this does not mean that it is 'all in your mind'. All illnesses, including CFS/ME, have physical, psychological, and social aspects.

5
Other associated conditions

People who are diagnosed as having CFS/ME may have other symptoms. A doctor may make other diagnoses (offer other 'labels') for these symptoms. These diagnoses may include one or more of the following:

- irritable bowel syndrome (IBS)
- non-cardiac chest pain
- fibromyalgia (FMS)
- pre-menstrual syndrome (PMS)
- hyperventilation syndrome
- anxiety and panic
- depression.

Poorly understood syndromes

There are a number of syndromes that are commonly diagnosed and have been fairly extensively researched, but for which the cause and treatment remains controversial.

Irritable bowel syndrome (IBS)

Problems with digestion and bowel functioning are common in the general population. They seem to be particularly common in people with a diagnosis of CFS/ME. Your doctor should be able to rule out treatable conditions such as coeliac disease (see Chapter 4) and other inflammations of the bowel.

The symptoms typical of IBS are altered bowel habit, bloating, and 'colicky' abdominal pains. As in CFS/ME, the diagnosis is made principally by exclusion of other medical causes of the symptoms. The cause is unknown. Dietary changes (such as adding roughage to the diet) sometimes help. The symptoms may, at least in part, be stress related. Learning to relax, to manage stress, and to reduce worry often helps.

Non-cardiac or 'atypical' chest pain and palpitations

Pains in the chest or an awareness of the heart beating are common symptoms. Because they suggest a problem with the heart, these symptoms can be particularly frightening. If you suffer from these symptoms, it is wise to see a doctor to ensure that they are not due to heart disease. Heart disease is common in our society and therefore needs to be excluded. Your doctor may wish to arrange tests such as an electrocardiogram and sometimes an exercise test. In most cases, however, particularly in younger people, the heart will be found to be healthy.

'Stress', anxiety and panic often cause these symptoms. Once a person has experienced chest pain, it can be made worse by worry about the symptoms themselves. After heart disease has been excluded, some people may require specific psychological help to manage these symptoms. The approach described in this book should also be helpful.

Fibromyalgia (FMS)

Where aches and pains are prominent without evidence of muscle or joint disease, a diagnosis of fibromyalgia (previously called fibrositis) may be made, especially if there are 'tender spots' in certain places on the body. FMS is so closely related to CFS/ME that it has been suggested that CFS/ME and FMS are in fact the same condition. They certainly overlap. Research into FMS has shown that the treatments of choice are similar to some of those commonly used for CFS/ME; that is, relaxation, graded increases in physical activity, and the so-called 'antidepressant' drugs such as amitriptyline (Trypizol or Elavil).

Pre-menstrual syndrome / tension (PMS / PMT)

Some women report a worsening of CFS/ME symptoms and increased irritability in the days leading up to their menstrual period. They may be given a diagnosis of PMS/PMT. A variety of treatments have been suggested for this syndrome. There is evidence that the so-called 'antidepressant' drugs, especially SSRIs (selective serotonin reuptake inhibitors) such as fluoxetine (Prozac), are effective for many with this syndrome (see Chapter 22). Exercise has also been shown to help. Recognizing that these are the most difficult days of the month can be useful to you so that you can pace yourself carefully through them. However, we suggest that you do not just focus on these days but also apply the more general approaches we describe *every day* and see how much they help.

Hyperventilation (over-breathing)

It has been suggested that hyperventilation is the cause of CFS/ME. However, studies have found that although some of the symptoms of some patients with CFS/ME may result from hyperventilation, it does not appear to cause all the symptoms. If you suspect that hyperventilation may be one of your problems it is worth discussing it with your doctor. He or she could help you to learn breathing exercises or you could be referred to a physiotherapist for similar help. This may reduce at least some of your symptoms. Hyperventilation also occurs in people who are suffering from anxiety and panic attacks (see below).

Fairly well-understood syndromes

There are several syndromes that can cause fatigue (and other physical symptoms) that have been well researched and are now fairly well understood. There are also well-established treatments for them. These syndromes include depression, anxiety, and panic.

Depression

It may surprise you to hear that depression is commonly associated with *physical* symptoms, not just emotional ones. These can include fatigue, muscle pain, and sleep problems. If symptoms of depression are present in addition to those of CFS/ME it does not necessarily mean that the illness is 'really' depression— but it does strongly suggest that treatment of depression will help you, and may reduce physical symptoms as well as emotional ones. Whatever else is wrong, it is better not to be depressed. Depression usually gets better if treated with antidepressant drugs or with cognitive behavioural therapy. The self-help approaches that are described in Chapter 22 are also likely to be useful for depression.

Anxiety and panic attacks

Worry, stress, anxiety, and panic attacks can all cause *physical* symptoms. They do this by activating the body's 'alarm system'—preparing it to fight or run away. This system includes the sympathetic part of the nervous system and the release of a hormone called adrenaline. Activation of this alarm system, such as occurs in anxiety and panic, causes a person to breathe more quickly, to have a faster heartbeat, and to tense muscles. Repeated activation of this alarm system can produce profound fatigue.

The physical symptoms of anxiety and panic can be frightening in themselves, especially if they lead the person to fear that they have a life-threatening disease (for example, chest pains suggesting a problem with the heart). This fear of disease has the potential to cause a vicious circle. The circle works like this: anxiety produces physical symptoms, the sufferer regards these physical symptoms as evidence of serious disease, and the fear of disease (or even death) leads to more anxiety and yet more symptoms. People who have severe anxiety and panic may require help from a doctor or psychologist (for drug treatment and/or specialist psychological treatment).

Controversial syndromes

There are other syndromes related to CFS/ME, the names of which not only describe the symptoms but also imply a cause. This makes them controversial, if the suggested cause is not generally agreed. These controversial syndromes include multiple chemical sensitivity (MCS), candidiasis (widespread infection with a yeast called *Candida albicans*), and hypoglycaemia (low blood sugar). Although there is no doubt that chemicals, *Candida albicans* infection, and hypoglycaemia can cause symptoms, research suggests that it is very unlikely that these are producing symptoms in patients with CFS/ME. We would therefore urge you to be very cautious about accepting these diagnoses or treatment based on them.

Multiple chemical sensitivity (MCS)

Those who believe in multiple chemical sensitivity as a cause of symptoms suggest that if symptoms appear to be associated with exposure to one or more chemicals, such chemicals are the cause. Although the reality of the person's symptoms is not in doubt, the suggestion that the chemical causes the symptoms remains an interesting but unproven idea. Those who make this diagnosis commonly advocate avoidance of many situations as treatment. This treatment is not based on sound evidence and is potentially harmful. Avoidance can improve symptoms in the short term but increase them in the longer term. It also reduces social contact and quality of life. It should not be undertaken lightly and we do not recommend it.

Systemic candidiasis

Candida albicans is a yeast, which can be a cause of vaginal discharge (thrush) and white sore patches in the mouth and skin. All of these can be treated safely by the use of anti-fungal drugs such as clotrimazole (Canestan or Lotrimin) or nystatin (Nystan or Nilstat). Some people have suggested that an 'overgrowth' of *Candida* in the gut can cause the symptoms of CFS/ME. This theory may sound plausible but it is not supported by evidence. The treatment following this diagnosis usually involves drastic changes in diet, the use of supplements and probiotics, and perhaps the prescription of anti-fungal drugs like nystatin. These treatments have adverse effects. The dietary changes can be difficult and interfere with adequate nutrition. The supplements recommended can be very expensive. Anti-fungal drugs can be toxic. We cannot recommend this form of treatment.

Food allergy and sensitivity

Some people blame illness on what they eat and some aspects of diet can lead to diseases. Many people with CFS/ME feel that certain foods worsen their symptoms for reasons that are not well understood. This is rarely because of a true allergy. Allergy is a relatively uncommon way in which food can cause disease. For instance, some people are allergic to certain foods such as peanuts. If you do get definite symptoms of allergy—such as tingling and swelling of the tongue and lips, wheezing, or rash—this is potentially life-threatening and you should see your doctor.

Whatever some therapists may say, there is no good evidence that CFS/ME is due to food sensitivity. If you feel better avoiding certain foods it may be reasonable to exclude them from your diet. But do be careful—excluding too many foods may put your nutrition at risk and can certainly reduce your quality of life.

Hypoglycaemia (low blood sugar)

Low blood sugar is a potential problem for people being treated for diabetes mellitus where the treatment may reduce the blood sugar more than necessary. However, there is very little evidence that other people have symptoms caused by low blood sugar. There is no good evidence that low blood sugar is a cause of CFS/ME. Taking excessive sugar with the idea of combating 'low blood sugar' is not justified and may cause weight gain.

What do I do if I have been given one of these diagnoses?

Discuss it with your doctor. If you also have CFS/ME, the main thing to recognize is that being given one of these diagnoses does not necessarily mean that you have more than one problem—rather, it is likely that each group of symptoms represents different aspects of a common problem. Which label you get given may to some degree depend on which specialist you see—a rheumatologist might use the label fibromyalgia, when a gastroenterologist might use the label irritable bowel syndrome. Furthermore, although there are specific treatments recommended for some of these conditions, they are all likely to be helped by the self-help approach we outline in this book.

If you have been given a diagnosis of CFS/ME you may have a number of symptoms. It may not be clear whether they are all part of CFS/ME or not. Your doctor or therapist may tell you that you have another condition. If this is one of the conditions we have discussed in this chapter, it is probably another aspect of the same problem rather than something new. The suggestions we make in this book are likely to be of use in helping you to manage any of these conditions, so do not let labels confuse you or prevent you from working to manage your symptoms. Some of the better-understood conditions such as depression, anxiety, and panic respond to specific medical and psychological treatment. If you think you have one of these you should discuss it with your doctor.

6

Research into CFS/ME

There has already been a great deal of research into CFS/ME. The aims of this research have been to find out the size of the problem in the population and the factors associated with it (epidemiology), to understand the causes (aetiology), and to find a test which will positively diagnose the condition (diagnostic test). Research is of course ultimately devoted to finding a cure. Research into treatment (clinical trials) is discussed in Chapter 8.

Before we go on to discuss what research has been done and is being done, as well as likely directions for future research, we need to give you a warning. It is essential that anyone with CFS/ME should have an appropriate degree of scepticism when reading about 'new research into CFS/ME', particularly research that is heralded as 'finding the cause of the illness', 'finding a diagnostic marker for the illness', or 'finding a cure'. The process of doing scientific research is a slow and difficult one. Progress in science is largely one of trial and error—much of what is reported is later disproved and it can be hard to know which finding will stand the test of time. There is a great deal of research published. It has been said that we could reduce the confusion by discarding half the published research—the problem is we do not know which half!

So before having hopes raised, read the following. These points may also be useful to combat over-enthusiasm for new findings and treatment amongst family and friends on your behalf!

- Before any meaningful research can be done, it is important that different researchers work out ways of ensuring that they are studying the same kinds of patients. Hence the importance of a definition of CFS/ME which has clear instructions on how to decide whether a patient qualifies for that diagnosis (see Chapter 3). In any published research it must be made clear exactly which patients the findings refer to.

- Beware of any research findings that appear in the media or popular magazines before they have been published in a reputable scientific journal. Before doctors and scientists can get research findings published in such journals they have to have their work reviewed by other scientists (peer review) and by the editor of the journal. This is a basic safeguard against faulty or misleading findings being published. However, it is not infallible. Even if something has been published in a journal, that does not necessarily mean that it is true. And, of course, some journals have more rigorous procedures and are more reputable than others!

- Even with this basic safeguard of peer review, any finding that cannot be repeated by other scientists with another group of patients is unlikely to be worth much. The field of CFS/ME is sadly littered with published observations (often heralded as 'breakthroughs') that have subsequently not been confirmed by other researchers. Most have later disappeared without trace.

- Association does not necessarily mean cause. Just because a chemical or some other measure is increased or decreased in people with CFS/ME does not mean that this is the cause of CFS/ME. There can be other explanations. In one famous study of another illness, a change in the urine that was thought to represent the chemical cause of that illness turned out to be an effect of the hospital diet!

- Scientific findings are often not clinically relevant. Even if they are true, many, if not most, research findings do not have any immediate relevance to the investigation and treatment of individual patients.

- Science is not just a laboratory exercise. Science is a method of finding the truth by carefully collecting and weighing evidence (as opposed to guess work, prejudice, or dogma). This discipline is as relevant to the clinical evaluation of patients and treatment as it is to the study of cells in a laboratory. Sadly, even some laboratory scientists may be less than scientific when they come to evaluate their favourite laboratory findings in patients (particularly if they stand to gain fame or money!).

Having outlined some of the limitations and hazards of research, we can tell you something about what has been found so far. We have also included books and published papers in our reading list that can give you more details of research into CFS/ME.

Research into CFS/ME in populations (epidemiology)

Epidemiology can tell us how much of a disease there is in the population (how many cases), what factors are associated with it, and what the outcome is for people suffering from that disease.

There has been a limited amount of epidemiological research into CFS/ME. How common it is found to be (its prevalence) depends on how a 'case' of CFS/ME is defined—and, in particular, how disabled the person has to be before they are accepted as a case. The rates found therefore vary. Reported figures are between 0.2% and 2% of the population. These studies show that CFS/ME occurs in all social classes but is more common in women—the reason for this is unknown. The peak age of onset is about 30 years but all ages can be affected.

The outcome studies available suggest that most patients do improve rather than deteriorate, and by 5 years after onset, half feel they have recovered.

Research into the cause of CFS/ME

This section is about what has been found out about possible causes of CFS/ME. When we talk about 'cause' we should explain that we mean by this both what might have started off the illness and what might be keeping it going (read more about this in the section on the three 'P's in Chapter 7).

There have been many studies into the causes of CFS/ME. These are summarized briefly under a number of headings:

Infection and the immune system

There has been a great deal of research in this area. Because many people with CFS/ME say that it started with a 'virus' infection, this has seemed an obvious place to start. One question is whether people who get any sort of infection are more likely to get CFS/ME; perhaps surprisingly, they do not seem to be. Another question is whether people who are infected with certain specific infections are more likely to get CFS/ME. The infectious agents studied include the Epstein–Barr virus (that causes glandular fever) and Q fever agent. There is some evidence that people who get these infections are more likely to go on to get CFS/ME, but how the infection does this remains uncertain. Although some virus infections may trigger CFS/ME in certain people, we do not have any good evidence at present that the symptoms of CFS/ME are caused by a persistent virus infection. Treating people with CFS/ME using the few drugs available that kill viruses does not seem to help them.

It has also been proposed that an alteration in the body's immune system could be responsible for the symptoms of CFS/ME. A good deal of work has been carried out to look for evidence of this. The immune system seems to be slightly abnormal in some patients with CFS/ME (but not all). However, the importance of these findings remains uncertain. The changes found are relatively small and can occur in other illnesses such as depression. It is not clear that they cause the symptoms of CFS/ME. However, there are links between the immune system and the brain (see below) that might yet turn out to be important. Research continues in this field.

Muscles

As so many people with CFS/ME report muscle pain and muscle weakness, researchers have looked at muscle function. The findings to date do not seem to indicate that these problems are due to a fault in the muscles themselves. Rather, it is more likely that the problem may be in the central nervous system and may be something to do with the way messages to and from the muscles are sent and received by the brain (see below).

The brain

The common symptoms of CFS/ME are fatigue, sleep disturbance, and poor concentration. There is also some evidence that people with CFS/ME find it more difficult to do complex mental tasks. These symptoms point to a problem with the brain. Sophisticated methods of looking at the structure of the brain with 'scans' (CT, MRI, etc.) have all been used to study people with CFS/ME. Most doctors believe that the structure of the brain is normal in patients with CFS/ME; that is, there is no evidence of brain damage. If there are no problems in the structure of the brain we might ask if the problem is in how it is working—its functioning. Other types of brain scan, such as SPECT (single photon emission computed tomography) and PET (positron emission tomography) can look at the functioning of the brain. Some of the studies that used these scans have reported a slightly lower blood flow (hypoperfusion) in certain areas of the brain (though different researchers have found this in different areas). These findings suggest changes in the demand for blood by certain areas of the brain because they are more or less active than usual. They do not, as some have suggested, indicate that blood vessels are blocked in CFS/ME.

Another way to find out about brain functioning is to do tests that tell us about the levels of different neurotransmitters (the chemicals that enable brain cells to talk to each other). Some studies have found these to be abnormal in some patients with CFS/ME. In particular, one area of the brain where these neurotransmitters may be abnormal is the hypothalamus. This is a small but particularly important part of the brain that controls hormones via the pituitary gland. There is some evidence that suggests that this system is not functioning quite normally in people with CFS/ME (see stress hormones below). There is also evidence that these changes may differ from those usually seen in people who are depressed (see below).

Stress

Stress is the name given to physical, psychological, and social pressures on a person that make them feel 'stressed' or under strain. Stressors can include such things as simple environmental factors, such as noise, excessive worry, or being badly treated by other people. Illness itself can be stressful. The symptoms of being under stress include fatigue, sleep disturbance, irritability, depression, and anxiety. Stress has major physiological effects on the body. In particular, it has effects on the nervous and hormonal systems, especially on the release of cortisol from the adrenal gland (see below).

Patients with CFS/ME commonly report suffering a period of stress prior to the onset of the illness. Does stress cause CFS/ME? There is some evidence that it may, in that an increase in life-stresses before the onset of illness has been noted. But stress can be the trigger for a wide range of illnesses and it is still unclear why some people get CFS/ME after stress whereas others do not. Stress may only be a cause in people who also have some other factor such as an infection. In summary, whereas most clinicians think stress is an important factor in many people, the scientific evidence for this is limited. More research is needed.

Stress hormones

When we are stressed—physically or mentally—our brain tells our adrenal glands to increase the level of cortisol in our blood. This is done by a part of the brain called the hypothalamus, which changes the chemicals released into the blood by the pituitary gland. This in turn controls output of cortisol by the adrenal glands. The whole system is called the hypothalamic–pituitary–adrenal (HPA) axis. People who have a faulty HPA axis (such as those with Addison's disease) often feel severely fatigued. It has been suggested, therefore, that it may be the brain's control of stress hormones that is defective in CFS/ME. There is some evidence for this but the abnormalities found so far are small. A group of people with CFS/ME may have *on average* a lower level of stress hormones than healthy people; however, this does not mean that this difference will be detectable in all *individuals*. Furthermore, the benefits of giving cortisol as a medicine to people with CFS/ME remain unclear.

Problems with the body clock—Circadian rhythms and sleep problems

People with CFS/ME commonly report disturbed sleep, most commonly broken and unrefreshing sleep and altered times of sleep. It seems obvious to suggest that poor sleep may lead to increased fatigue. There has been some research into the sleep problems experienced by many people with CFS/ME and whether these are the cause of fatigue. The results seem to indicate that although disturbed sleep and abnormal sleep/wake rhythms may contribute to fatigue, muscle pain, and poor concentration, they are not the basic cause of the illness. However, this is an area that may still turn out to be of interest, and research continues.

Changes in blood pressure—postural hypotension

It has been found that a proportion of patients with CFS/ME show an unusually large drop in their blood pressure when moving from lying to standing. This has been investigated by having the patient lie on a special table that tilts (a tilt table). Blood pressure and symptoms are monitored while the tilt table is moved from horizontal to vertical. There is a suggestion from these experiments that dizziness and fatigue are made worse in some patients when they stand up (and their blood pressure goes down). This finding is of interest and could be due to changes in brain function.

However, it is still unclear just how common this problem really is in people with CFS/ME and whether it is a cause of the illness or simply an effect of being ill—such as being less active.

The effects of inactivity

We all need rest but research has shown that too much rest can be harmful. Prolonged inactivity, even in fit persons, can itself cause fatigue and make it harder to be active. It can also have very profound effects on the body and mind, such as changes in blood pressure regulation leading to postural hypotension, changes in the body's ability to tolerate activity, changed temperature regulation, and actual physical changes in the functioning and the bulk of muscles. Some people with CFS/ME become persistently inactive and for them it is likely that inactivity contributes to their symptoms. Many others appear to become trapped in an oscillation between inactivity and activity. The effects of this oscillating pattern of activity are poorly understood. It would appear, however, not to help the body to regain its capacity for normal activity.

Depression and anxiety

Many studies have found that depression and anxiety are very common in people with CFS/ME. It has even been suggested that depression is the cause of CFS/ME. It is true that it can be very hard to sort out whether symptoms like fatigue, muscle pain, and poor concentration are due to depression and/or anxiety or to CFS/ME. However, this is not the same as asking whether depression actually causes CFS/ME. In fact, that is probably not even a sensible question. This is because both depression and CSF/ME are diagnosed purely on the basis of the symptoms a person has—to say that depression causes CFS is saying that symptoms cause symptoms!

Another way to look at this question is to ask whether the *causes* of CFS/ME are the same as the causes of depression. To some extent they probably are, as stress and the resulting changes in the functioning of the brain and hormone levels seem to play a role in both. In other ways they are probably not, as the actual changes observed in brain and hormonal function are different—for example, the stress hormone cortisol tends to be increased in people with depression but decreased in people with CFS/ME.

It is also reasonable to expect that the experience of CFS/ME could cause depression. If you have an illness over which you believe you have no personal control, it is likely to make you feel helplessness and hope-lessness about the outcome. A feeling of helplessness and hopelessness is, in turn, one of the recognized causes of depression. There are, therefore, a number of possible reasons for depression. A person with a diagnosis of CFS/ME may have symptoms of depres-sion and it can be hard to know which is which. In practice, the problem is easier. Depression can be treated, so if there is any doubt it is often wise to try a treatment for depression and see if it helps.

Patients' coping strategies and their understanding of the illness

There is evidence that people who believe very strongly that their illness is a disease caused by factors outside their control, and who deny the importance of psychological or social factors in their illness, have a worse outcome. A belief that the symptoms caused by activity are dangerous also seems to be associated with greater disability. These research findings could mean that these people simply have a more severe physical illness. However, that does not seem to be the reason. Rather, it seems more likely that this way of thinking about the illness leads people to cope in ways that do not encourage recovery—for example, by resting, avoiding any activity that seems to make symptoms worse, not getting treatment for depression, or not working on their rehabilitation.

The behaviour of other people

People are not simply individuals. They relate to and are influenced by the people about them—family, friends, doctors, officials, and those around them at work. These social factors can have an influence on how ill a person with CFS/ME feels and what they are able to achieve. There is less research into this aspect of CFS/ME, but most patients and doctors are aware of its importance. There is research into patients' experiences of CFS/ME that has illustrated just how difficult it is to manage any illness well in a climate of disbelief, particularly if that disbelief is coming from those close to you. If those around you do not accept or understand your illness, it can be much more difficult to cope effectively, and can add to your distress. You may find yourself with a need to demonstrate repeatedly to others just how bad you are feeling. Self-doubt may also creep in, fuelling premature attempts to 'behave normally'. (We talk about ways to explain an 'invisible illness' in Chapter 25.)

At the other extreme, excessive solicitousness or protectiveness by those close to you can be a real problem. Studies of patients with chronic pain have shown how well-meaning help from others can make a person more disabled than they need to be. Clinical studies suggest that, in some cases, a partner or parent may have found a role for him or herself in being a carer and so apply subtle and perhaps unconscious pressures on the sufferer to be dependent.

Finally, if a person has had to give up employment and exist on benefits or insurance payments, it can be difficult to make the switch back to working. Studies of other chronic illnesses, such as back pain, show that once people are off work for a long time, it becomes unlikely that they will return. That is probably because managing the transition from illness to working—especially if you would have to function at your previous level—can be very difficult.

Research into a 'test' for CFS/ME (diagnostic test)

A development of a test has great appeal. It would counter the 'all in the mind' accusation. It might make diagnosis easier and more reliable. But unless it leads to a treatment, its value would be limited. None of the findings listed above is sufficiently specific to this illness to function as a 'test'. If, as is suspected, CFS/ME is indeed caused by a variety of physical factors, it is likely that only a subgroup of patients would be positive on any one test. This would raise issues for those who test negative. Several tests have been suggested and others are being developed. At present there is no established test or 'marker' for CFS/ME.

Future directions

Where do we go from here? Probably much of the research being done will continue to explore many of the ideas above, using increasingly sophisticated techniques. There is likely to be more research attempting to differentiate between subgroups of the illness—finding out what the different types are and whether there should be different treatments for different subgroups.

Another potentially useful direction for research would be to study those factors that are common to all chronic illnesses.

What is clear is that the future focus of research is likely to be on the brain and the nervous system. On the one hand, the brain affects the function of the endocrine and immune systems. On the other hand, the state and functioning of the brain is affected by what a person thinks and does and by the behaviour of others. A focus on the brain might be what unifies the study of the mind and the body in CFS/ME.

Much research into CFS/ME has already been done. So far, research has produced as many questions as answers. It is important that CFS/ME sufferers should be sceptical about some of the published research and try to judge the soundness of the evidence. Current research is focusing on the brain; how reversible changes in the brain cause illness; and how social and psychological factors affect the brain.

7
Making sense of what we know about the causes of CFS/ME

Unfortunately, this chapter is going to be full of 'maybes'. In spite of all the research that has been done, there are few definite facts. No single cause for CFS/ME has been identified. In fact, most experts think that there are probably several routes into the illness and yet other factors keeping it going once it has begun. Over the years many researchers have enthusiastically pursued theories that they have hoped would be 'the cause'. To date, none of these has achieved general acceptance. Most researchers now believe that CFS/ME will ultimately be found to include a number of separate conditions. This means that not all people who have had a diagnosis of CFS/ME may have the same illness—so research suggesting a cause in some people with CFS/ME may not apply to you.

A way of thinking about cause—the 'three Ps'

It has been suggested that looking for a single cause, even in one individual, may be a mistake. Instead, it may be more helpful to look for a number of causes. Different causes may be more important in different people and within one person may play different roles.

These roles can usefully be grouped into three categories that are sometimes called the 'three Ps'. These are the factors that make an individual more likely to get CFS/ME (Predisposing), those that may trigger the illness (Precipitating), and those that may tend to keep it going once established—the obstacles to recovery (Perpetuating). This way of looking at the illness may be less instantly appealing than the idea of a single cause. However, it does have the advantage of opening up a much wider way of thinking about cause, which in turn offers more ways that an individual can be helped or can help him or herself.

Predisposing factors

Relatively little is known about the factors that make a person more likely to develop CFS/ME. Doctors working in specialized clinics may recognize some things as frequently occurring in their patients' medical history, but these factors do not occur in everyone. An overactive or striving lifestyle with inadequate time for rest and reflection leading to chronic stress has been suggested as one predisposing factor. A previous history of depression seems to make it more likely that a person will get CFS/ME. Stress over a long period may also predispose some people to getting CFS/ME. It seems likely that there may be some genetic factor as well. However, none of these factors is enough in itself to explain why one person develops CFS/ME while another similar person does not.

Precipitating factors

Why might people who are in some way vulnerable to getting CFS/ME go on to develop the illness? Many, but not all, people with CFS/ME report that their illness had a sudden onset, often following an acute viral-type illness. A virus infection may act as a trigger for the illness in some people. A severe emotional upset such as bereavement, an accident, an operation, or some kind of trauma may be a trigger in others. It is possible that it is a combination of these factors that is important.

Perpetuating factors

It is natural for anyone to feel a need to understand why they *became* ill, but in practical terms it is more important to identify things that are *keeping* them ill— whatever may be preventing a natural improvement or recovery.

These perpetuating factors are the most important. This is because they are the targets for treatments. They may be different from the precipitating factors. For example, a virus infection may have precipitated the illness but by a year later be gone—other factors are preventing recovery. The factors perpetuating CFS/ME are only partially understood and various theories have been suggested. None has so far been proved to be definitely true. However, in all chronic illness there is evidence that multiple factors perpetuate symptoms and disability. In CFS/ME these might include biological changes such as changes in the functioning of the brain and the HPA axis (see Chapter 6), psychological factors such as unhelpful thinking about symptoms, and social factors such as other people's lack of understanding of the illness.

A multifactorial theory of the perpetuation of CFS/ME

Although we do not know for certain what perpetuates CFS/ME, a combination of

1. evidence from research into CFS/ME,

2. evidence from research into related conditions such as chronic pain, and

3. our experience of listening to and helping people with CFS/ME

has led us to the following ideas. Many doctors and therapists (though not all) have accepted these ideas as our best understanding in our current state of knowledge. They have led to the development of useful treatments for CFS/ME such as cognitive behavioural therapy and graded exercise therapy. These are currently probably the most effective treatments for CFS/ME. These ideas are also the basis of many of the suggestions in this book.

This multifactorial theory suggests that:

1. many different factors (physical, psychological, and social) can perpetuate CFS/ME;

2. different combinations of factors may be important in different people;

3. these factors may interact to form vicious circles;

4. removing or reducing these perpetuating factors by breaking the vicious circles can aid recovery.

Factors that may perpetuate CFS/ME

The factors that can probably perpetuate CFS/ME include the physical, psychological, and social aspects of the illness listed below.

Physical

- abnormal brain functioning
- altered stress hormones
- sleep disturbance
- effect of inactivity
- possibly other changes such as immune activation.

Psychological

- unhelpful beliefs about the illness, such as 'there is nothing I can do'
- unhelpful coping behaviours, such as excessive rest, avoidance of activity, or oscillating level of activity
- negative mood such as depression and anxiety
- more general factors such as a lack of positive direction in life.

Social

- the failure of others to accept that you are ill
- a lack of understanding and support from others
- needing to prove all the time that you are unwell
- pressure from others to function normally

- overprotectiveness by others who do everything for you
- work stress making it difficult to return to a job.

Different factors may be important in different people

One of the observations made by anyone who has met many people with CFS/ME is that their symptoms and illnesses do not all seem to be identical. The careful assessment of individuals suggests that they may continue to have CFS/ME for different reasons. In some people inactivity is an important factor making them fatigued; in others it clearly is not. In others disturbances of sleep seem to be important and in yet others depression plays a role.

It is important to treat patients with CFS/ME as individuals and not to assume that the same treatment will work for all of them. The self-help programme we describe has many different parts. You are likely to find that some of these are more helpful to you than others. It may be sensible for you to consider which of the factors we have outlined could be important in perpetuating your symptoms and disability.

How do these factors interact to perpetuate illness?

The illness-perpetuating factors we have discussed may interact to form vicious circles. Some examples of these, with suggestions of how they can be broken, are:

- Your sleep is unrefreshing and fragmented. You feel tired. Because you feel so tired you tend to sleep during the day. You are also less active. Doing less and sleeping in the daytime tend to worsen the quality of your night-time sleep. And so on.

  Advice—improving the timing and quality of your sleep can help you feel better.

- If the changes in brain function make you more easily fatigued, you will be likely to reduce your level of activity, but you may keep making attempts to go on being active—and concluding that each time you try you only seem to make yourself feel terrible. You will understandably feel that activity is best avoided. A lower level of activity may perpetuate the brain changes that cause fatigue. And so on.

  Advice—a very gradual increase in activity seems to reverse the changes in brain function and help you do more and feel better.

- If you are unable to do what you did before, you will lack the sense of achievement and may become depressed. Depression makes you more fatigued. Fatigue makes you able to do less. And so on.

  Advice—effective treatment of depression can help you do more and feel better.

- Stress probably worsens the brain malfunction of CFS/ME. Being unwell is in itself very stressful. This is especially the case if others do not believe that you are really ill. You will probably feel that you should be doing more—and may even doubt your own symptoms. You may try to do what you did before and be unable to sustain it—or simply feel you are letting people down. All these things add to your stress and worsen the symptoms. And so on.

Advice—stress management can help you feel better.

Targeting treatment

Treatment is aimed at identifying and overcoming illness-perpetuating factors. Identifying any of the vicious circles we have mentioned and finding ways

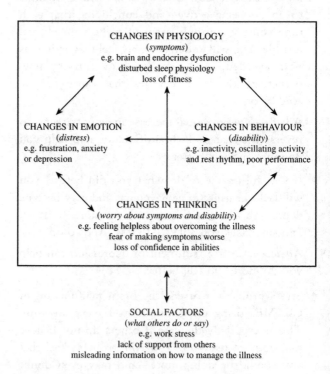

Figure 1 How the factors that can perpetuate CFS/ME can interact and produce vicious circles.

of breaking them will give your body a chance to recover naturally. You might like to trace examples of the vicious circles outlined in Figure 1.

Thinking, emotions, behaviour, and physiology all interact with one another. A change in any one can have an effect on the other three. Social factors can also have effects. It can be helpful, therefore, to think about how all of these things could be influencing you and your illness (and perhaps producing some of the vicious circles we have talked about). Once you have identified what applies to you, you could decide how you could break the circles.

It is unlikely that there is only one cause of CFS/ME. None has been found so far. It may be more useful to look at the 'three Ps'—Predisposing (what makes a person vulnerable), Precipitating (what triggers the illness), and Perpetuating (what keeps the illness going). The mixture of these factors probably varies between patients. The perpetuating factors could be physical, psychological, or social—and probably a mixture of all three. The trick is to identify those that are important in any particular case and to work towards overcoming them.

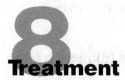

8
Treatment

The bad news is that at the present time there is no cure for CFS/ME; the good news is that there is a lot that can be done to manage symptoms and disability and to speed recovery.

The first requirement of someone suffering from such symptoms and disability is for sympathetic understanding both from their doctor and from those around them. Unfortunately, this is not always forthcoming. For reasons we talked about earlier, some doctors feel uneasy with a CFS/ME patient. Because they can find no 'physical' cause, they may dismiss the symptoms as being caused by some 'mental' state. Such a dismissal can be distressing and frightening for a patient. Luckily, medical opinion is changing and more and more doctors are recognizing CFS/ME as a 'real' illness, even if its causes are not yet understood. Even if your initial contact with your family doctor does not seem to be particularly helpful, you can work towards a better relationship with your doctor. We talk more about this in Chapter 26.

Many medical treatments have been tried in CFS/ME. Unfortunately, few are supported by good evidence that they help. We will go through a list of treatments, summarizing the evidence for each. Remember, however, that one of the main points of this book is that there is a great deal you can do to help yourself.

Research into treatments (clinical trials)

It is important to understand that before a treatment can be recommended, it must have been properly tested. The 'gold standard' of such tests is a randomized controlled trial (RCT). In an RCT patients are allocated randomly to one of two groups; one is given the new treatment and the other another treatment (sometimes a placebo or an inactive pill, sometimes the current usual care). Allocating patients randomly makes sure that the patients in both groups are similar—both in ways that can be measured and in other ways that might not be obvious.

RCTs are often done 'blind', which means that neither the patient nor the doctor giving the treatment is told which treatment a given patient has received. The reason for this is that it prevents the effect of enthusiasm for the new treatment influencing the results. It is normal in any such trial for as many as a third of the patients receiving the placebo to report an improvement, so if the active drug is effective it needs to be substantially more successful than that.

To be a good trial it should be as large as possible to include a wide range of patients and minimize the possibility that any difference (or lack of difference) in the outcome is simply due to chance.

It is also important that when an RCT is repeated in a different centre, similar results are obtained. This is another way in which we can be confident that any benefit the new treatment seems to offer is real.

Finally, the long-term effects of the treatment should be monitored to see how long the benefit lasts and to ensure that no harmful effects become apparent that were not revealed in the short-term trials.

Any new drug treatment for CFS/ME would have to go through this process before it could be licensed, which could take up to five years. Sadly, even if an effective drug were found very soon, it would not be generally available for some time.

No treatment—wait and see

Before considering any treatment, it is worth considering whether it is better to do nothing—to simply wait and see. The advantages of doing this is that no money will be spent on worthless treatments and no adverse treatment effects will be suffered. The disadvantage is that you will not receive the potential advantage of more active approaches. While for some illnesses a wait and see approach is often appropriate, we are concerned that too many people with CFS/ME have accepted this without being aware of alternatives. These are discussed below.

Drug treatments

Medications may be prescribed either to ease a particular symptom or in the hope of dealing with what might be the underlying cause of the condition. As new research findings emerge so new treatments based on them are tried. So far none of the drug treatments has shown much overall success, although some of them have been reported as having limited success for some patients.

Anti-viral drugs

As so many patients believe that their illness began with a viral infection and some of the symptoms feel 'viral', this seemed a reasonable area for treatment. However, a trial of the anti-viral drug acylovir did not produce encouraging results.

Drugs to help the immune system

Various drugs acting on the immune system have been tried. The chemicals produced by the immune system, immunoglobulin and gammaglobulin, have been given as a drug without much success. The latest drug in this range to be tried is a chemical called ampligen. At this time it is only being used by a few doctors (almost always in a research setting) and it has the major drawback of being extremely expensive. It may or may not prove to be helpful, but there is still very little long-term data available. The latest information about this drug is not encouraging.

Drugs to treat low blood pressure

Drugs have been used to treat this condition in patients who have been proved to have this problem. Preliminary results have been encouraging, but only for those patients with the problem of low blood pressure.

Cortisol

As we mentioned earlier, there has been research indicating that some CFS/ME patients have a lower level of cortisol than normal (as opposed to those suffering from depression who often have a higher level), which may perhaps be something to do with the HPA axis not functioning quite normally. This has prompted trials of giving cortisol as a drug (in the form of hydrocortisone). At this time results are somewhat mixed. There are certainly hazards from taking these steroid drugs long term. At present this treatment cannot be recommended.

Other hormones and mineral supplements

We are aware that some practitioners advocate a variety of hormones and mineral supplements as treatments for CFS/ME. There is no evidence, how-ever, for the effectiveness of these and we recommend that they are avoided.

Antidepressants

The word antidepressant is used as an 'umbrella term' for a group of drugs. One of the actions of these drugs is to improve depressed mood. However, the name antidepressant is something of a misnomer. These drugs actually have widespread actions on the func-tioning of the nervous system. One might argue that it would be more accurate to call them 'brain tonics'. Given that there is now a consensus that the symptoms of CFS/ME are most likely to originate in malfunc-tioning of the central nervous system, these broad spectrum 'brain tonics' are likely candidates to help.

These agents tend to normalize problems with appetite, sleep, pain, and energy, as well as mood, so it is probably worth trying them. For example, if you have problems with disturbed or unrefreshing sleep it would be worth trying one of the sedative tricyclic antidepressants such as amitriptyline (Trytizol or Elavil) or trazodone (Molipaxin or Desyrel). These drugs are also good for pain. The newer SSRI drugs (see Chapter 22) such as fluoxetine (Prozac) are good for mood but less effective in improving sleep and in reducing pain.

If your mood is low and your doctor suspects that you may be depressed, it would certainly be worth trying antidepressant medication for this. Depression is something that can and should be treated. Having CFS/ME is bad enough without being depressed as well. We talk about this and antidepressants in general in more detail in Chapter 22.

Analgesics

Pain can be one of the most distressing symptoms of CFS/ME, so it is not surprising that people seek ways to reduce or eliminate it. On the whole, any painkillers are better used from time to time rather than on a regular basis. You may get more benefit from a low dose of a suitable antidepressant, which can be used regularly. We talk about the pros and cons of various analgesics and other ways of managing pain in Chapter 17.

Sedatives

If you have difficulty getting to sleep or if you wake often during the night it may be tempting to ask your doctor to prescribe a sedative. Such drugs may be helpful if used for just a short time but, unlike antidepressants, they can produce quite serious problems if used for longer. Some of these drugs can be addictive and they can also become less effective in time. We talk about other ways of managing sleep problems in Chapter 15.

Complementary/alternative therapies

Many people with CFS/ME make use of these therapies. We go into the subject in more detail in Chapter 31. They range from the well-established complementary therapies that your own doctor might suggest to some alternative therapies that have no scientific basis and could be dangerous. Many of the alternative therapies involve vitamin or mineral supplements or the use of herbal remedies, although there is very little proof that these are necessary or do much good. If you find something that is helpful to you in some way, then use it. But do be cautious. All active treatments—complementary, alternative, and conventional—have risks and side-effects. We would argue that your recovery or improvement is probably more likely to depend on what you do for yourself in the way of self-help than on any specific therapy you receive.

Non-drug treatments

So far, attempts to identify a drug to treat CFS/ME successfully have had limited success. However, there has also been research into non-drug treatments. This has produced rather more encouraging results. Such treatments have been shown to be a considerable help to patients with CFS/ME, if not a cure.

This seems as good a moment as any to bring up the subject of a referral to a psychologist or a psychiatrist as such therapies are often administered by them. Many people with CFS/ME feel deeply affronted if their doctor suggests such a referral. They may take it to mean that their doctor does not believe that they have a physical illness. They may resent bitterly the suggestion that emotional problems are causing their illness. Such feelings are understandable. However, it is worth considering the benefits that such a referral might have, particularly if the psychologist or psychiatrist is knowledgeable about CFS/ME:

- Psychologists and psychiatrists are able to give their patients much more time than a busy family doctor can spare. For many of the people we have talked with, this was their first opportunity to tell their whole story and discuss *all* their problems. You might find this an extremely helpful process.

- In many places there are no medical consultants specializing in CFS/ME. Often the only possible referral is to a consultant specializing in just one aspect of your many symptoms. A psychiatrist may be available who is prepared to look at the whole illness.

- Any illness is likely to produce some emotional problems. Talking these over with someone understanding can make them easier to deal with.

- Depression can be a real and understandable problem for people with CFS/ME. Although most cases of depression are treated very successfully by family doctors, psychiatrists may be more experienced at treating severe depression. They may also be more knowledgeable about tailoring an antidepressant programme to suit an individual patient.

- A psychiatrist can often provide the gateway to the therapies such as cognitive behaviour therapy and graded exercise therapy that we discuss next.

Not all psychiatrists or psychologists will be naturally sympathetic to the patient with CFS/ME, but try and get the best from your doctors (this is a topic discussed further in Chapter 26).

Cognitive behaviour therapy (CBT) and graded exercise therapy (GET)

Both of these therapies involve therapists and patients meeting regularly to discuss illness-related problems and to give guidance in self-help. Cognitive behaviour therapy (CBT) gets its name from the combination of looking at the ways patients think about their illness (cognition) and the way they cope with it (behaviour). The therapies are based on the theory of illness perpetuation described in Chapter 7.

CBT and GET have certain similarities. Both aim for rehabilitation using a gradual change in behaviour carried out as a collaboration between patient and therapist. They have both been proved to help some patients to some degree. However, both therapies have attracted some criticism from patient organizations. Much of this criticism results from misconceptions (see Chapter 9) or from experience of poorly implemented forms of CBT and GET in which patients have been told to increase activity at a faster rate than they felt comfortable doing. Good CBT and GET is simply 'help with self-help'. There is no forced change in behaviour or activity—simply guidance and encouragement to the patient to try things out and draw their own conclusions about the value of these changes. We talk about these therapies in much more detail in Chapter 32.

At this stage of medical knowledge, doctors cannot prescribe a drug that will cure CFS/ME. With all the research that is being carried out, there is a possibility that this situation may change, but it is not likely to happen in the near future. Putting your life on hold, while waiting for a miracle drug, is not likely to help. You do have options. Probably the best option today is to work on increasing what you can do and on managing your symptoms positively. You can do this using the self-help techniques that we talk about in Section 2. These self-help techniques may be easier to do if you have help from a person or therapist who can guide you. However, there is much you can do yourself by simply using this book.

9
Some myths about CFS/ME

Before reading this book you may have gathered other information about CFS or ME. This will probably have come from things other sufferers have told you, or from magazine articles and books, some of which could have been written some time ago. You may well have been told some things as 'facts', which may be only partially correct or, worse still, not true at all. Some of these 'myths' may get in the way of you managing yourself and your illness in the best way. Here are some of the 'ME myths' we have heard about from sufferers:

- *The only treatment for CFS/ME is rest, rest, and more rest.* This is very far from the truth. Everybody needs good-quality rest. However, research has shown that too much rest is not good for anyone. Like too much food it has harmful effects in the longer term. The best way forward is combining rest with building in small amounts of daily activity that are very gradually increased.

- *People with CFS/ME should never take antibiotics.* Indiscriminate use of antibiotics for any ailment is not a good idea for anyone. However, there is no reason to avoid them when needed. For instance, if you developed an abscess under a tooth, that would certainly be an appropriate time for antibiotic treatment.

- *Anaesthetics are bad for people with CFS/ME.* This is often said, but it is based on no real evidence. Any operation is likely to be tiring and stressful, especially if you are feeling ill to start with, but there is no good evidence that the anaesthetic is more harmful if you have CFS/ME. Do not allow yourself to be put off having essential treatment.

- *If you have CFS/ME, you have a problem with Candida overgrowth in your intestines.* There is no good evidence for this idea. It is a myth.

- *If you are not trying alternative therapies you are not really trying to get better.* If you try the self-help techniques we advocate you will certainly be doing your best. (What is more, they will cost you very much less.) There is no alternative therapy of proven effectiveness in CFS/ME—whatever people may claim.

- *You should be using large amounts of dietary supplements.* Again, this is something that has not been proved by proper research. It is a myth.

- *You should have any dental fillings containing mercury amalgam removed.* There is little evidence that mercury amalgam fillings have much effect on anyone. There is no good evidence that they cause or maintain CFS/ME. The process of removal could be very expensive, potentially hazardous, and certainly would be very stressful and tiring. It would probably do you much more harm than good.

- *Until a drug cure is found, there is nothing that can be done to help a person with CFS/ME.* Although there is as yet no drug therapy to cure the condition, research has shown that the sort of techniques described in this book can make a difference. Such techniques can be even more effective if practised with the help of a knowledgeable therapist.

- *Cognitive behaviour therapy (CBT) and graded exercise therapy (GET) are harmful for people with CFS/ME.* They are not. These therapies, if properly implemented, are simply ways of helping the patient to increase activity *at their own pace.* Forced increases in activity should not be part of GET or CBT. Most patients with CFS/ME who have tried and persevered with CBT and GET have been able to do more as a result. As with all active treatments there is a risk of side-effects and a small number of patients who have been treated with GET and CBT report feeling worse afterwards. There is, however, no evidence that they have been harmed. You could read Chapter 32 in which we describe what is involved in CBT and GET treatment for CFS/ME and then judge for yourself.

It is not only fellow sufferers who can spread myths about CFS/ME. Doctors can do so too. Some medical recommendations reported back to us are also myths:

- *CFS/ME is not a real illness. It is all in your mind.* CFS/ME is a real illness and involves both the body *and* the mind.

- *You should push yourself through it.* Cautious increases in activity after stabilizing your level of activity can be helpful; rushing into increased activity is generally not.

- *You need exercise therapy. Go to your local gym and get to work.* Graded exercise therapy is something very different from that. It involves cautious and structured increases in activity.

- *You are just depressed.* It is possible that you are depressed. 'Just' is hardly an appropriate word as depression is serious and can cause physical symptoms. You can be depressed while also suffering from CFS/ME.

- *There is nothing that can be done to help with CFS/ME. You will just have to wait for a natural recovery.* You can do a lot to help yourself in the process of recovery. You do not have to wait helplessly.

As you get more experienced in managing your condition, you will be more able to distinguish myths from reality on the basis of your own experience. Do not let myths discourage you from gathering more experience of your illness by trying out the self-help techniques that we discuss in the next section.

10
Summary

As you can see from all we have written in this section, there is a shortage of real facts about CFS/ME and some of the associated conditions. No one is certain exactly what causes these illnesses. There is no diagnostic test for the illness and there is no medical treatment that has been proved to help everyone. However, we do know quite a lot about what stands in the way of recovery from CFS/ME and how to overcome these factors. There is a great deal that individuals can do to help themselves. We will talk about this in the next section of the book. To sum up what is *known* about the best way of dealing with CFS/ME:

- Do not put your life on hold waiting for the 'magic bullet' of a medical treatment. You do not have to wait to be *made* well—instead you can concentrate on all the things that will help you *get* well and you can work on improving your quality of life meanwhile.

- Treat what can be treated. For instance, if you suffer from depression, see if you can get that treated. If you have severe pain, consider the careful use of painkillers. Anything that reduces the overall burden on you will be helpful.

- Rest but keep active. Try to get your sleep and activity into a comfortable and regular pattern.

- Once you have stabilized your routine, try very gradual increases towards planned targets.

- *Managing* yourself and your illness is the key to success.

We hope that you will read the next section of this book with an open mind. What we suggest is based on proper research and on years of experience of advising people with CFS/ME and then seeing the results of that advice. You have nothing to lose by trying out these techniques and we believe that you have a lot to gain.

Section 2

The idea of self-help

11

Introduction to self-help

The fact that there is as yet no single identified cause or proven medical cure for CFS/ME does *not* mean that there is nothing that can be done about the condition. For a start, your doctor may be able to help you with symptom relief and perhaps refer you to other health professionals who can assist you in your quest for improvement.

More importantly, though, there is a great deal that you can do to help yourself. Our bodies are very good at healing themselves if we give them a chance. We now know quite a lot about what you can do to help (or hinder) your body's natural healing (based on both research evidence and clinical experience). This section of the book will outline all the things that will help to make you feel better and to give you the best chance of being able to regain a normal life.

We are going to start by looking at what you can do in an effective way to manage your life and your illness by adopting what might be called 'health-promoting behaviours'. Later we will look at how your emotions can have an effect on your condition. Finally we will suggest some practical ideas about ways in which you could make your life easier or more pleasurable, which would also be an aid to improvement.

As you read through this section, you may feel that it is a bit daunting. What we suggest may seem to require too much discipline and too many changes to the ways in which you behave and manage your life. Most people have these reservations at first, but find that it gets easier and that the benefits make the discipline and changes worthwhile.

It will certainly make a difference if you can get all the support possible from those around you—from a partner, family, or friends—by helping them to understand what you are doing and why. Perhaps you could get them to read this section of the book if not all of it. Alternatively, we recommend a patient information booklet in the reading list which gives a summary of what we suggest.

How to do it

Depending on where you live, you may be able to attend one of the specialist clinics that offer treatment for people with CFS/ME and suggest such behaviours. If you do not have access to one of these, this section will outline what such a service would advise so that you can treat yourself. It will be easier for you if you can find someone knowledgeable who can support you in what you are doing and give you advice and encouragement. Many doctors, occupational therapists, psychologists, and counsellors are able to do this. Alternatively, you might have someone close to you who could give you help and encouragement. However, it is possible to do it on your own.

When to start

The earlier in your illness that you can begin this active illness management the better, but there is no reason to assume that if you have been ill for some time this sort of thing is not for you. We know of many people who have been ill for a long time who have made significant improvement when they changed the way they were managing their illness. Even if you are very severely ill, there is a possibility of improvement, though it may be a very long slow process. Patience and discipline are going to be important (sorry about that!).

12
Balancing rest and activity

This is one of the most important things you can do to help yourself. Although we can describe general principles, you will need to work out a personalized 'programme' of rest and activity to suit you and the way you are now. After all, *you* are the expert on *you*.

The 'roller-coaster'

Too many people with CFS/ME live on a roller-coaster, alternating bursts of activity with periods of doing much less—the 'boom or bust' or 'push–crash' problem. They do too much one day, feel much worse as a result, and are then able to do much less for the next day or two. After resting during this time they wake up feeling much better and immediately try to catch up, do too much, and crash again. This does not help their bodies and usually adds to their feelings of frustration. Many people with this pattern of activity end up being able to do less in total because of the times when they can do so little. It is often said that CFS/ME is a very fluctuating condition but in our experience it is sometimes the patients' behaviour and activity that fluctuate, leading to exacerbation of symptoms. Pacing is a way of avoiding this problem.

Pacing

'Pacing' means alternating time-limited periods of activity, both physical and mental, with periods of good-quality rest. Your aim should be to stop *before* you get exhausted. Getting a bit tired will not do you any harm, but getting exhausted on a regular basis is not helpful. The best idea is to start at a level well within your capacity, even if that means doing rather less to begin with. The principles of pacing will help you whatever your level of activity. You are likely to find that stopping while you are still only a bit tired, rather than keeping going until you are exhausted, will mean that you need much shorter periods of rest to recover from the exertion. This pattern of activity is also likely to help you feel better.

Mental activity can be as tiring as physical activity, so something like sitting and watching television does not count as real rest. Try to alternate using your body and using your mind with intervals of rest between each activity.

Pacing may mean changing your way of life considerably and accepting that you often have to stop something before you have finished it, take a break for a rest, and then come back to it later. You definitely should *not* work on the 'I've started, so I'll finish' principle. Pacing requires discipline. In Chapter 20 we

look at what can make that discipline more difficult—
'what gets in the way of being sensible'. Wait until you
have read that chapter before you decide that it is all
too difficult for you. In Chapter 27 we talk about
'budgeting' your energy expenditure, which can also be
a help.

Keeping an activity diary

It may help if you keep a brief diary for a *few* weeks in
which you record activities, timings, symptoms, and
feelings. We have included some suggestions on doing
this in Appendix 2. After you have kept a record for a
while, you will probably be able to spot patterns, such
as the swings between doing too much and doing too
little. It is typical of CFS/ME that the effects of getting
too tired do not necessarily show up until the next day
or even the day after. You need to anticipate this. The
information from this diary will help you plan out a
'programme' of balanced rest and activity. A structure
to your day, with targets set and achieved (however
small they may need to be), will help to give you back a
sense of control in your life.

Pleasure and satisfaction

When you are planning your programme, it is important to include things that give you pleasure or
satisfaction. Pleasure is one of the things that is really
good for your body and your spirit. It is so easy to
believe that, because you have got CFS/ME and cannot
do all the things you once could, you cannot enjoy

yourself. That is not necessarily so. It is worth exploring other ways of enjoying yourself that fit in with your present circumstances. We talk more about this in Chapter 27.

Rewards

Many people find it easier to stick to a pacing programme if they do not make it too rigid and if they give themselves rewards for good pacing.

Jake found that he could be much more successful in his pacing if he gave himself a treat at the end of a week in which he had managed to stay disciplined. He allowed himself a long-distance call to a good friend, partly as a reward and partly to report how well he had done.

Where are you now?

Accept where you are now. What can you comfortably do now (not just on a good day) and then repeat the next day? Be honest with yourself. This is your starting point. We are often asked 'How long should my periods of activity be?' Each person is different, so there is no absolute rule. Your activity diary should help you decide what is an appropriate period and what is 'going on too long' for each activity.

Be consistent

Your 'programme' should be something you can keep up in a *consistent* way. Consistency really is vital even though it may mean that, for a while, you have to do rather less. However, many people are surprised to find that by spreading out their activities (over the day and over the week) they end up being able to do rather more.

Sue used to do her housework in one burst in the morning, only stopping when she was completely exhausted. The rest of the day she felt very ill as well as frustrated by not having been able to achieve all she wanted. Then she tried the experiment of limiting herself to 15-minute chunks of activity. Between these chunks she sat down, relaxed, and had a rest. At the end of the first week she was astonished to find that she had achieved rather more and yet was not feeling so tired and ill.

You may find that it takes some time to adjust to this new way of doing things. You probably will not get it right immediately and will need to keep working at it. Most people find it takes time to change. You do not need to be too rigid about your programme either. There are bound to be times when things outside your control get in the way. Do not worry about that; just come back to the programme again as soon as you can.

Make increases gradually

Later on you are likely to find that it can be possible to increase the amount you do, either by making your periods of activity just a little longer or by doing things more often during the day. However, it is vital that when you make these sorts of changes, you do it in a very restrained and gradual way. We talk more about this in Chapter 19.

Sticking to a consistent pattern of physical and mental activities, both during the day and during the week, with intervals of rest between activities, is one of the best things you can do to help yourself. Plan out a programme for yourself and make sure that it includes things that give you pleasure or satisfaction as well as the necessary chores. This consistent programme could well reduce some of your symptoms and start you on the path towards improvement.

13

Relaxation and calm breathing

Relaxation is one of those words that can mean different things to different people. What we mean in this context is not just 'taking it easy'. We mean letting go of physical tension in all your muscles. Tensed-up muscles use energy that you cannot afford to waste.

Deep physical relaxation and calm breathing are both things that will help your body. In the previous chapter we talked about periods of good-quality rest between activities. You will rest much better if all your muscles are relaxed. It may take time and practice to learn how to do this. There are tapes and books available that can help you in this (you will find some suggestions in Appendix 4), but you can start it on your own.

When and where

Choose a time when you are not going to be disturbed. Get yourself really comfortable, whether lying down or sitting in a chair that supports your neck and arms.

Relax your muscles

Some people find that if they first tighten up the part they want to relax it helps them recognize the difference between tense and relaxed, but others find this too tiring. Experiment for yourself and decide what suits you. Start by taking a few calm, slow breaths. Now think about one hand. Tighten it up into a clenched fist for a moment and then let it go. Feel the difference between tight and loose. Think about your hand, wrist, and arm getting warmer and heavier. If someone were to take hold of your cuff and lift your wrist, you would not help them by using your arm muscles and, when they let go, your hand would flop down again. In your mind move round your body, letting go of the tension in all your muscle groups in the same way. Your shoulders and neck are an important area to concentrate on. Think about your face too. If you are frowning or your teeth are clenched, it is much more difficult to relax. Work towards a calm, peaceful expression.

Relax your breathing

Calm breathing is important. Some people with CFS/ME breathe rapidly or erratically, particularly if they are feeling anxious or panicky. Learning good breathing techniques and practising them regularly will be a very good idea. Your aim should be to be able to use all your lungs—letting your ribs and your diaphragm do the work—rather than just the top of your chest. Ask for help from your doctor if you find this difficult.

Relax your mind

Your relaxation periods are *not* times for thinking too hard or for worrying. Try to switch off from anxious or unhappy thoughts by thinking about something else, something peaceful and happy. Trying to make your mind a blank does not work. Some people find it helps if they visualize a special place, a sanctuary all their own, concentrating on all the details of sight, sound, smell, etc. Others find the techniques of meditation extremely helpful in giving them a period of calmness and rest. Experiment with what works for you.

After relaxing

When you come to the end of your relaxation period, do not leap up immediately. Give yourself a little time to take a few deep breaths and to stretch a little. Think about how a cat stretches before it gets up.

Practice

Do not feel that you have to master this skill right away. Spend time on it and practise it regularly. As you get better at it, you will find that you can switch it on whenever you need it—and not necessarily just while lying down. Periods of relaxation and calm breathing during the day will help to reduce pain and the 'flu-like' feelings. It is certainly one of the things that will help you in both getting to sleep and coping with periods of wakefulness during the night. It is also a technique that will help you deal better with stress.

Possible problems

To begin with you may find that you do not enjoy relaxation or find it comfortable. Some people tell us that they notice pain or malaise more when they are not being distracted from it by activity (this does not mean that the symptoms *are* worse—just that they are more noticeable). If you have been in the habit of being busy, switching off may make you feel a little guilty at first. It gets easier and more enjoyable with practice.

Being able to relax both your body and your mind is a skill that many people need to learn and practise. Regular periods of relaxation will help you feel better and give you better quality rest. Good breathing habits will help your body.

14

Appropriate exercise

Rest

You may well have found that doing nothing for a day or two reduces your symptoms and so believe that more rest is the answer. However, although we all need reasonable periods of good-quality rest, too much rest does not help our bodies. It can lead to muscle weakness, stiff joints, poor circulation with postural hypotension (loss of blood pressure control causing dizziness on standing up), and back problems. It also causes loss of motivation and poor concentration.

Research for the American space programme has shown that prolonged rest—even for periods as short as two weeks—can cause these changes, even in fit young people.

The periods of relaxation that we discussed in the previous chapter are *not* the same as prolonged rest. Short periods during which you relax your body and mind are very beneficial; *prolonged* rest (lasting days and weeks) is not.

Are you suffering from the effects of inactivity?

Some of the problems and symptoms you are experiencing now could be because you have got out of condition since you became ill. (We do not mean by this that deconditioning is the only reason you are still ill.) For instance, spending a lot of time lying in bed can make you feel weak and worsen back pain. It really will help your body if you can keep it moving, even if all you can manage is a small amount at intervals during the day. Little and often works well. Try to build appropriate periods of physical activity into your 'pacing programme'. If you are uncertain where to start, you could ask for a fitness assessment from a physiotherapist, who would be able to plan out an exercise programme appropriate for the way you are now.

Getting fitter

Try not to be overambitious. Forget what you used to be able to do before you were ill. Just concentrate on what suits your body *now* and work out what you can do comfortably and for how long. Warm up with gentle stretches and stop when you have completed what you planned. Do *not* carry on until you feel too tired to continue. A small amount done regularly is going to do you much more good than doing too much one day and being too tired to do anything the next day.

Here are some suggestions about how you can help yourself:

- *Bending and stretching exercises*—joints that are not used get stiff, muscles that are not used can get shorter and weaker, so very gentle exercises will help to avoid problems. Start very gradually. You can do gentle exercises even while lying down. It is sometimes easier to do exercises in warm water. If there is a swimming pool within easy reach, you could try using the learner pool (which is often at a higher temperature) at a quiet time.

- *Walking*—this is one of the best forms of exercise, even if you can only manage a small amount. (You could walk indoors if the weather is bad, though it can be rather boring.) Two short walks morning and afternoon are better than one longer one that leaves you exhausted. You will probably find that by splitting your walks into smaller chunks you will be able to walk further in total. You may only be able to manage a few paces at first, but even that will be a good start.

- *Swimming and cycling*—if your condition allows it, these are both good forms of exercise if done gently and in moderation. Pace yourself carefully, always stopping before you get too tired.

- *Posture*—if you are feeling tired and weak, it is very tempting to slouch or sit in a slumped position. Think tall! Good posture is much kinder to your body.

Once you have achieved a level of exercise that you can do in a consistent way, you can begin the process of increasing it very gradually. This is something we discuss in more detail in Chapter 19.

> Keeping your body moving will help to avoid the dangers of getting out of condition and will keep you in the best shape possible. Aim for small planned amounts, done regularly, that do not leave you too tired. Once you have found a stable level of exercise that you can tolerate, the next step is to plan a gradual increase.

15
Improving your sleep

People with CFS/ME often find that their sleep patterns have changed. At the beginning of their illness they sometimes sleep much more. Later on they may find that they have difficulty getting to sleep or that they may wake during the night. Often, even if they have slept, they still wake up feeling tired. Good-quality sleep, at normal times, is something we all need, so it is worth looking at all the ways that you can get back to this.

Getting to sleep

You can experiment with all the things that help you get to sleep, such as establishing a calm routine that leads up to bedtime and relaxing when you get to bed. The period just before sleep is *not* the time for thinking about problems—which will make it much harder for you to settle down. Many people find it helpful to set up a specific 'worry time' earlier in the day. If you find yourself anxious about some problem while you are trying to get to sleep, tell yourself that you will think about that tomorrow during your worry time. Avoid alcohol and caffeine-containing drinks for a couple of hours before bedtime—they may make it harder to get to sleep.

Getting back to sleep if you wake in the night

If you wake during the night, try to stay calm and relaxed. Build up a collection of gentle, pleasant things to occupy your mind. That way you will still be getting rest and you are more likely to fall asleep again. Relaxation techniques (as in Chapter 13) will help you get the most rest possible while you are awake.

Worrying about not sleeping is almost guaranteed to make it much harder to get back to sleep. If you really cannot sleep, do something else like reading or listening to music until you begin to feel sleepy again. Then go back to bed—and to sleep!

Establishing a pattern

You need to establish regular times for going to bed and for waking. Research among people with CFS/ME into the way the body's rhythms work show how important this is. Many people have noticed the similarity between the symptoms of CFS/ME and those of 'jet lag'.

You may need to re-establish such a regular pattern and to avoid sleeping at other times. If you have slept badly during the night, it is very tempting to sleep longer in the morning, but this is not a good idea. The sleep patterns of some people with CFS/ME can get chaotic, even going as far as sleeping most of the day and being awake most of the night. This makes it difficult to take part in normal social activity and can worsen the illness. You may need to use an alarm clock or a timed radio to help you wake at a regular time. You can always rest later in the day if you need to.

If you are feeling very tired it may seem reasonable to have naps during the day. This may be the right thing for you, but it might make it more difficult to get to sleep at night. If you want a daytime nap (and if it will fit into your schedule), try to have it at a regular time (like a 'siesta' after lunch). Experiment to see what works best for you.

Using sedatives

If these simple 'sleep hygiene' methods are not enough, you might want to consider taking one of the several types of sedative medicine. Those most commonly prescribed are benzodiazepines, such as temazepam. These are safe and effective but can interfere with the quality of sleep and can also be addictive. The antihistamines, such as promethazine (Phenergan) or cyproheptadine (Periactin), also have a sedating effect.

It is better to avoid using sleeping pills on a regular basis because you may become dependent on them (unlike antidepressants). They may make you sleep longer, but it will not be very good quality sleep. However, you could talk to your doctor about using them for a limited period.

A good alternative is to take a low dose of a sedative 'antidepressant' drug such as amitriptyline (Tryptizol or Elavil) or trazodone (Molipaxin or Desyrel) an hour or two before you go to bed. Such drugs are not just prescribed to help mood, they have a lot of useful effects for improving sleep and helping with pain. At this low dosage they are very unlikely to have any unpleasant side-effects.

> Improving your sleep pattern is an important part of your overall strategy for helping your body to recover. It is worth experimenting to find what helps. Try to stay relaxed if you do find it difficult to go to sleep or if you wake during the night. Worrying about not sleeping will only make things worse.

16
Getting the best from your food

If you are feeling very tired and unwell it can be all too easy to neglect yourself, going for the easiest options in meals and eating at odd hours, but a good diet is important for health. Regular, good-quality meals should be part of your plan for giving yourself the best chance of improvement. Try to get back into the habit of having meals at consistent, normal times—breakfast, lunch, and supper. Some people feel better if they do not go for too long between meals. If you are one of them, then including small, healthy snacks between meals can be a good idea.

A normal healthy diet

What should you be eating? Basically, what you should be aiming for is a well-balanced diet of good-quality food including all the different food groups. Many people prefer a low-fat, low-sugar diet. However, you should try to include a wide variety of food. The following are generally accepted as part of a healthy diet:

complex carbohydrates (wholemeal bread rather than white); pulses (beans, lentils, etc.); plenty of fresh fruit, salads, and lightly cooked vegetables; good-quality low-fat protein; milk, and cheeses; eggs; liver (but not if you are pregnant); and oily fish (such as tuna and mackerel).

We are deliberately not suggesting a special diet for people with CFS/ME—just the sort of good food that makes up a normal healthy diet and which doctors would recommend for anyone. Beware of restrictive diets suggested as treatment—there is no evidence that they help and they may cause harm.

Food supplements

Your aim should be to get all the nourishment you need from what you are eating. You may have read that if you have CFS/ME you should be taking massive supplements of minerals and vitamins. There is no evidence at all that this is necessary. Supplements like these can be very expensive. Nourishment is probably more easily absorbed from food than from pills. It can be dangerous to take too much of some vitamins (such as Vitamin A) and for most others our bodies simply excrete what they do not need, so you could end up with most of what you have paid for disappearing down the toilet.

Alcohol, tea, and coffee

Many people with CFS/ME find that alcohol makes them feel worse. If you are one of them, you may wish to limit your intake or even to cut it out. Other people also choose to reduce the amount of tea, coffee, and cola they drink (all of them contain the stimulant caffeine). This may be helpful.

Weight change

Being overweight or underweight can be a problem. If you are taking much less exercise because of your illness and yet are still eating the same amount as before you became ill, it is very easy to put on weight. Comfort eating can also lead to weight gain. Carrying too much weight will only add to your fatigue. Similarly, it is not helpful to lose too much weight. If you have a problem with weight, talk to a doctor or dietician and get advice on a diet that will keep your weight stable.

Depression can produce problems both in weight loss and weight gain. Some people who are suffering from depression lose their appetite. Some of the drugs that are used to treat depression can have a side-effect of increasing appetite and weight; others reduce them. Discuss this with your doctor if he or she is prescribing an antidepressant for you.

Tired of cooking (or tired by cooking)?

Eating well does not mean that you have to spend a lot of time cooking. You can get all the nourishment you need from very simple food. For instance, a sandwich made from wholemeal bread, cold meat or tinned tuna, with a tomato or some fresh fruit and a glass of milk is a perfectly healthy meal.

Keeping diet and food as normal as possible

One general rule that applies here is that it is better to do things as normally as possible unless there is a good reason not to. You do not need to change from your previous eating habits unless they included a lot of junk food or irregular meal times. If so, this might be a good moment to change to a regular, healthy diet which would be something of benefit to you for the rest of your life. Enjoying what you eat is one of the basic pleasures in life, so try to eat healthily and happily.

A good, well-balanced diet with meals at regular times is an important part of your strategy for improvement. Give your body all the nourishment it needs for health and recovery. Supplements of vitamins and minerals are not necessary for most people with CFS/ME. Enjoy your food.

17

Coping with pain

For many people, pain is one of the most difficult and distressing symptoms of CFS/ME. We often hear patients say, 'I could cope with just being tired. It's the pain that makes life so difficult.' It may be a constant background to your life or it may be intermittent, perhaps made worse by overactivity. Being in pain can be very tiring and can often interfere with normal sleep, so anything you can do to manage your pain—to reduce it or to lessen its impact—will be a help to both your body and your mind. Different people experience different kinds of pain, which can include:

- muscle and joint pain
- headaches
- sore throat
- abdominal pain.

We can offer you some suggestions for strategies for managing your own pain but, as with most of what we suggest, you will have to experiment to find what works for you.

Check out that it is all due to CFS/ME

Do not assume that every symptom is due to CFS/ME. Discuss this with your family doctor or your consultant. Make sure that other conditions that could cause pain have been considered and treated.

Consider whether some of your pain could be a consequence of lack of activity or poor posture. This is likely to be an added factor if you lead a very sedentary life or spend a lot of time in bed. Muscles that are not used get weaker; joints get stiff like rusty hinges. When they are used they hurt. You could try a minimal exercise routine to stretch and strengthen your muscles and to keep your joints mobile (as in Chapter 14). Good posture may help to prevent some of these problems.

Relaxation

Pain is made worse by muscle tension. Sometimes the pain is actually caused by it. For instance, some headaches are a result of tension in the neck and shoulders. Try the effect of relaxing in response to pain instead of tightening up against it.

Distraction

Pain is always more of a problem when we are focusing our attention on it. The more we concentrate on it, the worse it is likely to become. Distraction is a good technique to help reduce your awareness of your pain, even if you can only keep it up for a few minutes at a time. Any moments of respite are to be welcomed. Once you have got yourself relaxed, try moving on to focusing your awareness on something else. Experiment to find out what works best for you. It could be music or a talking book, or just thinking of something pleasant and relaxing. Sometimes concentrating on a bit of your body that is *not* hurting, even if it is just your little finger, can help.

Splitting the sensation and the message

This sounds complicated, so let us explain what we mean. Before you became ill, pain was often a danger signal. It could mean that something was going wrong and was often a cause for quite reasonable alarm. However, in CFS/ME you can be in pain without it meaning that there is anything dangerous going on. We tend to be conditioned by our previous experience and beliefs, however inappropriate they may be today, so that pain means danger and is frightening. You may well be afraid that pain means that you are getting worse, that you have caused yourself permanent damage, or that you have some life-threatening condition. We so often hear patients saying things like 'I know it sounds silly, but could such-and-such a pain mean that I could have heart disease/cancer/a brain tumour ... ?' You are not alone if you sometimes have thoughts like these.

Fear is a distressing and demoralizing emotion and it is exhausting too. It is bad enough hurting without suffering fear as well, so it is worth looking at the meanings you give to your pain, the labels you put on it, and checking on their accuracy. The more you can reduce the feelings of fear and resentment of pain, the easier it will be for you and the better it will be for your body. Fear and anger are stressful and stress often makes CFS/ME worse. Tension caused by these emotions can make your pain worse. You may need to get medical reassurance that you are not suffering from some dangerous condition; you may need to talk through your feelings of anger and resentment that you are hurting so much. Anything that helps in that way will be good for you and make the pain easier to cope with.

Other techniques

It is worth trying out all the things that help just a little. Do you hurt less if you are warm? Maybe a hot-water bottle in the right place will help or an electric blanket in your bed would make a difference. Does a warm bath make you feel better? A bath does not have to be only for washing—you could just relax and enjoy it.

The right kind of massage can sometimes help. You need to experiment to find what works for you. Sometimes a very light, delicate stroking of the skin above the sore spot can be nice and a distraction from the pain. Perhaps you could train a partner or a friend to do massage for you, if you cannot afford professional sessions.

Some people find that acupuncture can be effective for their particular kind of pain, though the relief may not last.

You may find that visualization can help. Some people can form a picture in their minds of their pain.

If you are one of them, you could experiment with trying to change the picture into something less aggressive (like changing an image of a tiger into one of a gentle kitten). If you think of the pain in a colour, you could try changing that colour to something softer and more friendly.

Painkillers

Like all medicines, painkillers (analgesic medication) have advantages and disadvantages. It is worth trying other strategies of managing pain, such as we have outlined earlier, rather than relying on just using such drugs.

Analgesics can help relieve pain, but in the longer term they can become ineffective and even addictive. There is evidence that prolonged use of analgesics can make headaches worse. All painkillers have some side-effects and people with CFS/ME seem to be particularly sensitive to them. Pain is very individual, so what helps one person may not help another. However, if you find something that works for you, even if you only use it very infrequently, it can make day-to-day pain easier to manage. You do not have to feel 'I have to bear this for ever.' Almost anything is easier to cope with if you know you could have moments when you could choose not to have to cope. One word of warning—a period of relief from pain can sometimes make you lose sight of your pacing programme.

There are various drugs that seem to give *some* relief to people with CFS/ME, but unfortunately there is no one drug that removes pain altogether or works for everyone. Some that are worth trying are:

- Soluble aspirin or paracetamol (not marketed in America) can sometimes give some relief, but they can have side-effects of gastric problems or liver problems if used excessively.

- Anti-inflammatory drugs such as ibuprofen (Brufen or Motrin) can sometimes help with pain in muscles and joints, but again they can have side-effects of gastric problems.

- As with sleep problems, a low dose of the so-called antidepressants such as amitriptyline (Tryptizol or Elavil) used on a regular basis can help with pain (whether or not you feel depressed). They are often used in Pain Relief Clinics for a variety of conditions causing pain. They are not addictive.

Opiates and drugs containing codeine are better not used on a regular basis. They can cause constipation and can interfere with sleep. They also have the major problem that they can be addictive.

Pain can certainly be a problem in CFS/ME, but there are ways in which you can lessen its impact. The self-help techniques we outline in this book can reduce pain. In the longer term, pain usually recedes with your general recovery. In the meantime you could experiment to see what helps now. It is generally better to avoid opiates and drugs including codeine. Experiment with the techniques we have outlined and see what helps you.

18
Difficulties with memory and concentration

One of the symptoms of CFS/ME that can cause great distress and can be very worrying is that of difficulties with memory and concentration. This is something that is very often reported by patients. It is quite normal to have these problems, but it must be stressed that it does *not* mean that there is any permanent brain damage. These problems will get less as your health improves. Research has shown that the degree of difficulty in things like short-term memory and concentration vary to some extent with your level of fatigue and with how ill you are feeling. Although these problems can be infuriating (and at times extremely inconvenient), they are not something to fear. Fretting about them could hold back your improvement.

What sort of problems do patients report? A common one is difficulty in reading, not necessarily because of eye problems (although they may be there too) but because it is hard to remember what happened earlier in the book. Another common problem is difficulty in finding the right word, or using the wrong word, which can be very disconcerting both for the sufferer and for those around them. Problems with memory mean that we often hear of people going into a room to do something and then finding that they cannot remember what it was. Concentration is often more difficult when you are tired.

Helping yourself

There is a lot you can do to help yourself, both in propping up a faulty memory and in doing small things to maintain cognitive function:

- Cut down on what you absolutely have to remember. Do not try to remember anything that you could write down.

- Use lists; write yourself notes. It can be helpful to use a notebook or something like a Filofax, so you know where you have made the note—you can waste a lot of time and effort trying to remember on which scrap of paper you wrote the information!

- Try to build up rituals and routines to help you remember things—such as always putting the car keys in the same place immediately you come into the house.

- Give yourself a few moments before you do something to get it clear in your head.

- Take time to consider what causes you the greatest difficulty and then think about practical ways to make things easier.

With something that really does need to be remembered, you can experiment with different ways of learning it. Writing it down, saying it out loud to yourself, using word association, and so on, can all make something easier to capture.

If you have difficulty concentrating, try doing the things that require concentration in much smaller 'bites'. Do a small amount, have a rest, and then come back to it later. Cut out distractions like noise or conversation. Choose a time of day when concentration seems a little easier to do the demanding tasks. One of the tasks that people with CFS/ME often find the most difficult and stressful is filling in official forms. Allow yourself to tackle them slowly, perhaps just doing one page or section a day. Forcing yourself to go on until it is finished will be very tiring and will probably mean that you do it much less efficiently. A warning note—putting off the difficult task will often mean that you face a deadline and then need to do it in a hurry. Try to start in good time.

Keeping in practice

It is also well worth keeping in regular practice with the things you find difficult. If you give up bothering with something because it is difficult, it is likely to get worse because you are out of practice. To a degree, it is a case of 'use it or lose it'. Your brain needs exercise as much as your body. To give just one example, if you often have difficulty finding the right word, crossword puzzles can be useful brain exercise. You do not need to do all of a puzzle, but just trying a few clues of the simplest puzzle will keep you in practice at retrieving the right word.

Difficulties with memory and concentration are quite common in CFS/ME, but they do not indicate permanent damage. Use every technique possible to make life easier for yourself. As your condition improves, these problems will get less. Keep on using your brain, even if it is difficult to do so.

19

A gradual increase in activity

There are two stages in this self-help programme. The first is to stabilize your activity and to look at all the other ways in which you can help your body, such as relaxation, better sleep, good diet, and pain management. Once you have put into practice some of the things we have talked about in the previous chapters and have adjusted to a level of physical and mental activity that you can manage each day, you can move on to the next stage. This is to start increasing your activities *just a little*.

You may decide that you would get a better quality of life if you concentrated on increasing your physical activity. In Chapter 14 we discussed the kinds of exercise that are helpful for someone with CFS/ME. You could start with just a small amount of some of these (perhaps only five minutes to begin with) and then go on to increase the time by a minute or two in gentle stages. This is the sort of approach that is used in the graded exercise therapy (GET) that we discuss in Chapter 32.

However, you may find it more helpful to think about increasing your general activity, looking at *all* the things you do—physical, social, and mental—and increasing them slowly and carefully. Some people find it easier if one week they concentrate on a small increase in some physical activity and the next week on some mental activity (while maintaining the physical increase). You do not need to increase all your activities simultaneously.

When you first start this increase it is very important not to be overambitious. For instance, if you are at present comfortable doing one particular thing for ten minutes, you could try the experiment of increasing it to eleven or twelve minutes (instead of doubling it as some people do). Another way would be to do it for six minutes, but then repeat it later in the day.

You may perhaps feel that by suggesting this sort of thing we are implying that you are lazy and are not doing enough. We certainly are not suggesting any-thing of the sort. Up till now you have probably been as active as seemed possible, but perhaps in the wrong sort of way.

Reluctance to try increasing activity

You may be tempted to say, 'I've tried this sort of thing before and it didn't work. It made me much worse.' Perhaps you were too ambitious or had not managed to get your pattern of activity consistent before you tried increasing it. You have nothing to lose by trying this experiment as long as you do it carefully and cautiously.

If you were previously very active, the increase in activity you are planning now might seem too small to be useful—you might even think that it is pathetic. Tell yourself that every journey begins with a single step—and compare your achievements with what you have been able to do since you have been ill, not with what you could do before!

If you have a very severe form of the illness, you may find it hard to believe that any increase in activity could be possible for you. We assure you that we know patients who were almost totally bedridden who have improved their condition by trying this kind of approach. It may be necessary to start with something very small, perhaps something as restrained as sitting up in bed for five minutes once a day and then increasing it to six minutes. That would be a beginning that could lead on to other things.

Setting targets

It is worth thinking about some very definite targets. Instead of thinking 'I'd like to be able to walk much further', try to replace that vague concept with something much more specific like 'I'd like to be able to walk to the park and back.' Then think about building up to that distance in stages over several weeks, or longer if necessary. Similarly, you can consider targets for mental activity and again build up to them in stages. You may find it helpful to give yourself a period of total relaxation immediately after each activity. Activities that involve both physical and mental exertion are likely to be doubly tiring, so be cautious about those at the beginning. Do try to build in pleasures as well as chores.

What to expect when you start

Do not be alarmed if your symptoms increase a little. That is completely normal. As long as it is only just a little and it does not last for more than a few days, you do not have to worry. You will not be doing yourself any harm. The usual pattern is that after a little while the body adjusts to this increased level of activity. Wait for a week and see if your symptoms ease off. Stay at this level for a week or two and then make another increase, but again one that is not too ambitious. If your increased symptoms persist, you may have made too big an increase. Slow down a little, wait for a bit, and then try again but with a smaller increase. Some-times you may need to stay at a certain level for two or three weeks before moving on again. If you get a cold or some other infection or if you get unavoidably exhausted, you may have to ease off for a while and then start increasing again when you feel a bit better.

NB: This gradual increase in activity has been proved to be the way through to a significant improvement for many CFS/ME patients.

However, there are various pitfalls along the way and it is worth warning you about them. If you know what to expect, it will be much less scary:

- You are likely to feel a bit worse when you start this sort of programme. You are not doing yourself permanent damage if you get a mild increase in symptoms. You just need to adjust to a new level of activity. This sort of programme has been tried out in many CFS/ME clinics and has been proved to be safe and to work. Do not give up just because you feel a little worse, even though it may be very tempting to think that you should go back to resting more.

- At a time when you are about to start another increase, you again may feel a bit worse, but this is likely to be due to feeling a bit nervous about it.

- If things are working well, you may be tempted to go ahead too fast, do too much, too soon, and crash. Taking things slowly without being too ambitious will be much more successful in the long term. Do your best to stay disciplined.

- Life can get in the way. You may have unexpected demands on your time and energy—a minor crisis, an unplanned visit, or a birthday. Just let it happen and then go back to your programme later.

- Improvement never happens in a straight line kind of way. You are bound to have times when you feel worse for no apparent reason. Do not be cast down by this or believe that it means that the programme is not working. Stick with it and wait for things to improve again.

This kind of gradual increase in activity may take quite a time to achieve significant results. It depends very much on your particular version of CFS/ME and on how long you have been ill. Do not despair because it seems that improvement is not happening as quickly as you would like. If you keep going, there is a very good chance that you will achieve a very much better quality of life, even though you may not get back to quite the state you were in before you became ill.

This sort of approach to treatment has been validated by proper research trials as well as by clinical experience away from research. It may not be a cure, but it has been proved in many cases to lead to a significant improvement in condition. It is certainly worthwhile making your own trial of it, even if you have to do it very slowly and cautiously.

Getting someone to help you

It can be very helpful to have someone working with you while you do this kind of programme. You may be able to find a health professional experienced in this sort of thing who can supervise your progress, discuss the problems you encounter, and encourage you to persevere. If you cannot find someone like that, you may be able to involve a friend or a relative, though it should be someone you really trust. Reporting your progress can be a real incentive. However, it definitely is possible to do it on your own, though probably you will need to move at a slower pace than if you had back-up.

Once you have achieved a pattern of consistency in your life, you could try the experiment of making cautious and controlled increases in both physical and mental activity. Setting goals for such increases and working carefully towards them is helpful. This approach has been proved to help many patients.

20
What gets in the way of being sensible?

You may decide that a pacing programme is a good idea, but it is very likely that you will find that sticking to it is not that easy. You will probably find that things get in the way—some coming from outside pressures, but some coming from your own beliefs and emotions. Clinical experience and research show that identifying the things that stop you pacing yourself as well as you could is extremely important in this kind of self-help programme. When you know what these barriers are, you can look for ways round them.

We can tell you of some of the most common things that get in the way of being sensible and suggest possible ways of getting round them, but you will need to recognize and identify what particularly applies to you. It may help if you keep a diary for a while, recording what you are doing, what you are thinking, what is happening at the time, and what the results are (see Appendix 2). If you can catch your fleeting thoughts just *before* you start doing something or at the moment when you decide to go on doing it for longer, it is likely to give you far greater insight into what pushes you into overactivity. You may be surprised to find that some of your motives for doing or not doing things are not very reasonable.

Doing too much

Most people are driven by imperatives—'oughts', 'musts', and 'shoulds'—often going back to childhood. If you think about yourself, you might be able to recognize some of your own. Typical ones can be: 'If you have started something, you really ought to finish it', 'You must try to do better than that', 'You should be getting on with things instead of just sitting around doing nothing', or 'If you aren't nice to people they won't like you.' You might even be able to hear the adult voice who said that to the child you used to be and challenge that voice as not being appropriate today.

Typical thoughts that you can begin to recognize as danger signals could be ones like: 'I'll just do a bit more and then I'll rest', 'I know I'm tired, but I do want to get this finished', 'People will think I'm being a wet blanket or selfish if I don't join in their plans', 'I'm tired of being sensible', or 'I must look after my family in the way I used to.'

So here are just some of the things we have heard about from other sufferers. Thinking about these may give you some guidelines, but you will need to recognize the things that specifically get in *your* way.

Pressures of just surviving

For a lot of people with CFS/ME—those living on their own, mothers with young children, people with unsupportive families, those struggling to keep on with a job—just doing the minimum to keep going can make overactivity almost unavoidable. It can help if you can stand back and look at all that you believe needs doing and consider whether *some* of it might not be absolutely essential. It might be possible to restructure the way in which the essential is done, breaking tasks down into smaller bites, and stopping for a rest between each one.

Lack of authoritative management advice

It is much easier to pace yourself and to 'sell' this idea to others if you can say, 'I am pacing myself in this way because my doctor tells me it is essential', rather than just, 'I have found from experience that this is the best way of managing my illness.'

Nevertheless, if what you do say is said with total confidence, it is much more likely to be received with belief and acceptance. Building up your confidence in your own judgement and expertise is vital.

Other people's expectations

It is only too easy to get sucked into doing too much by what you believe other people are expecting from you. It is worth considering three things:

1. Are your ideas about their expectations accurate? Could you check up on what they really do expect?

2. Are their ideas unreasonable or inaccurate? Could you communicate with them better, so that their ideas are more realistic?

3. How important is it to you to fulfil their expectations? Do you really need to please them if they are being unrealistic?

Your own model of a 'good person'

We all have an internal model of what a 'good person' is and does. Trying to match up your activities with this model when you are unwell is more than likely to lead you into doing too much. Your model may have suited you before you were ill (though it might have been one of the things that led you to overdoing it even then) but does it fit in with the way you are today? Could you change it for something more appropriate to your present circumstances, perhaps by thinking about your value from 'being' rather than from 'doing'?

Sharon felt that she ought to be doing more for and with her children. She felt that she would be a bad mother if she looked after herself instead of concentrating on them. After a while, though, she came to see that she was of value to them by just being there, able to listen to them when they needed to talk, and that if she pushed herself into complete exhaustion she was able to do less for them. Being good enough was better than trying to be perfect!

Being a perfectionist

This can be one of the things that really does get in the way of being sensible. If you still believe that anything you do has to be done to a very high standard, you are likely to push yourself far harder than is appropriate for the way you are now. You could try to look at the advantages and disadvantages of being a perfectionist. Why do you need to be so hard on yourself? What is wrong with being average? Are you still trying to prove something to someone from your childhood? Are you imposing standards on yourself that you would not expect from someone else in your position?

If you find it hard to shift from being a perfectionist, you might try telling yourself that the pacing programme takes priority and concentrate on doing that in the very best way possible.

Wanting more of a rare pleasure

If your life is restricted by illness it is very tempting to prolong a rare pleasure—'This is lovely; I want more of it *now*'—and so move from allowable fatigue into sheer exhaustion. Try to remind yourself that by stopping in time there is a much better chance of having pleasure tomorrow, rather than feeling very unwell.

Impatience

It can be very easy to slip into the trap of wanting to get something finished and out of the way and so keep on with it too long. Again, try to remind yourself that stopping in time will give you a greater chance of achieving things later. You can always come back and finish it when you have had a rest.

A desire to catch up on things after a bad spell

If you have had a time when your CFS/ME has been worse and then find yourself a bit better, it is very easy to leap into overactivity in sheer relief at feeling better. You may think of 'better' as a chance to catch up on all the things that have had to be left undone. Try to hang onto the belief that discipline is just as important in the good times. In fact, it is probably even more important.

Pride

Many people find that pride gets in the way of good pacing. They resent asking for help or feel that they would be less of a person if they dropped their standards. You might consider the difference between self-respect and pride. Self-respect is important; pride is not.

Getting carried away by an activity

When you are doing something absorbing, it can be very easy to go on too long and only notice rather too late just how tired you have become. Setting yourself time-limits is a good idea. Work out how long you can do a particular activity before getting too tired and try to stick to just that length of time. You could use a kitchen timer or an alarm clock to remind you when you have done enough. You can always come back to the activity later when you have had a rest.

Doing too little

So far we have only mentioned the factors that can lead to doing too much, but doing too little can sometimes not be sensible. We do *not* think that most people with CFS/ME do too little all the time. A more common picture is of a mixture of sometimes doing too much but, at the same time, doing less of some things that might be possible. It can be very helpful to think about what you avoid doing and why you avoid it. These are some of the reasons we have been told about.

Fear

CFS/ME can be such a bewildering condition, particularly if you have not been given authoritative guidance about how to manage it, that it can be difficult to be certain how much you can safely do. It can be tempting to avoid activity for fear of making yourself worse. We hope that this book will help you understand more about what is possible and safe.

If you did something and felt very ill afterwards, you can quite justifiably feel nervous about trying it again. However, it could be that you did too much of it or you did it at a time when you were already tired from doing something else. That activity might be within your capacity now if you timed it better or did it for a shorter time.

Most people with CFS/ME have one particular symptom that they dislike or fear more than the rest of the package. They are likely to be very dubious about doing anything that seems to provoke that symptom. It is always worth remembering that none of the symptoms are in themselves dangerous. It may help if you can change your thinking from 'This symptom is dangerous' to 'I don't like this symptom, but I don't have to fear it.'

Wondering what other people will think

You may well be nervous that if other people see you doing something out of the house they will disbelieve your illness. You may feel that they will think something like 'If he/she can do *that*, they can't really be that ill.' You may need to be prepared to explain that this is a rare pleasure and that other people do not see the times when you need to rest. We hear of people being frightened that if they are seen doing something even slightly active they may have their benefits withdrawn. These are likely to be inaccurate beliefs and worth challenging.

The effort of motivating yourself

There may well be things that you need to do or would like to do that would be possible, but the effort of getting organized to do them can seem to be too much bother. This can be particularly true if your mood is low. It is worth reminding yourself that doing them is likely to make you feel better—maybe not physically, though that is possible, but that it would give you a sense of achievement.

Doing things in the same way as before you were ill

There are likely to be many things that could be possible for you to undertake if you could tackle them in a rather different way. Forward planning and lots of advance preparation might make something possible that you have written off as not for you now. We talk more about this in Chapter 27.

Looking at what you are getting right

So far we have talked about the things that are likely to push you into not managing yourself as well as possible and suggested that you identify the factors particular to your own situation. However, another approach to good management is to identify the times and the circumstances when you get the balance between rest and activity right. Recognizing your successes and building on them is a very good idea.

Pacing yourself—doing enough but not too much—is a central part of your strategy for improvement. It really can help if you spend some time looking at all the things that get in the way of this. At each stage of your illness you may need to think and rethink about what gets in the way of being sensible.

Equally, you could benefit from identifying the times when you pace yourself well, so that you can build on your successes.

21

Improving your mood

Introduction

In the previous chapters we discussed some things you can do to help yourself in a practical way. In these next chapters we will look at the emotional aspects, which can be just as important.

We are well aware that many people with CFS/ME have to cope in a climate of disbelief. Their own doctor, their family, or their friends may suggest that their illness is somehow their own fault—that it is due to emotional problems or their inaccurate beliefs about their condition. In extreme cases they may even be told that they are not really ill—they only think they are. That can make it very difficult to admit to having emotional problems, which is very hard as *any* illness can produce such problems. Even if you do find it difficult to discuss such problems with most other people, it will certainly help if you can find someone safe to confide in. At least admit them to yourself.

Mind and body cannot be separated. Emotions and moods have a physical effect on the body and what happens to the body has an effect on mood. This is true of *any* illness, not just CFS/ME. Anything that you can do to improve your mood or to deal better with such emotions as loss, anger, frustration, and fear can be an important part of your programme to help yourself. Keeping worry, anxiety, and stress within reasonable limits will take some of the pressure off your body.

Mood

Having an illness like this can be a very depressing and frustrating experience. It is hardly surprising if you often feel in low spirits. One of the recognized symptoms of the illness can be mood swings (what doctors sometimes call emotional lability). You may find that you cry much more easily or get irritated by small things that would not have bothered you before you got ill. Often, getting too tired can push you into low spirits.

As in any long-term illness, you are likely to have times when you experience feelings of loss, anger, fear, or frustration. At times these feelings may seem overwhelming, but with practice they can be managed. Anything you can do to lift your spirits will be of value. It may help if you can find someone who feels able to listen when you need to talk about what is happening to you. It often works better if that person is someone like a counsellor or a friend with whom you are not emotionally involved—talking about these sorts of things to a partner or a close relative can often end up with both of you distressed.

Loss

You may grieve for the person you used to be before you were ill and for all that that person could do then. You may feel a sense of loss for some of your hopes for the future. We have spoken to many people who mourn these losses just as strongly as they would the death of a partner or a close friend. Talking about it will probably help, particularly if you can find someone to talk with who understands about bereavement.

Anger

Anger can be a very damaging and fatiguing emotion, though very understandable in the circumstances. Many people with CFS/ME feel enormous anger at their doctors for not being able to help them more or for not seeming to take their illness seriously. They often get very upset by other people not understanding what is happening to them. They may feel resentment at the poor support they are getting from those close to them (sometimes quite justifiably). This is a stage of illness that most patients go through, but it is important to move on from it. You do not want to get stuck in angry resentment. Improving your communication skills will probably reduce some of the areas of friction. We talk more about that in Chapter 25.

Fear and anxiety about the future

It is not surprising that you sometimes feel afraid of what is happening to you and what it might mean for your future. One thought to hang on to is that although CFS/ME can be extremely unpleasant and debilitating, it is *not* life-threatening. We hope that if you try some of the techniques we have suggested earlier, you will begin to feel a little better and so become more optimistic about the future. There is life after CFS/ME, even though it may be hard to believe that now. Allow yourself times when you think constructively about your fears, but do not dwell on them all the time.

Frustration

Frustration is a totally understandable emotion in the circumstances. There is so much you would like to do that seems impossible now. You may be able to find ways in which you can do just a little more of what you want, particularly if you can break it up into smaller 'bites'. We talk more about this in Chapter 27. The more you can work on finding ways round the problems, the better you will get at it, and the less frustrated you will feel. In Chapter 20 we talked about perfectionism getting in the way of being sensible. If you can accept slightly lower standards, even if just for now, you are likely to feel less frustrated.

Feeling depressed

Depression is one of those words that can mean very different things to different people. At one end of the scale it can be used to describe a feeling of low spirits or a temporary feeling of misery, but at the other end it can describe a persistent mood of deep despair. Many people with CFS/ME experience transient low mood and misery (often associated with being overtired after doing too much). Managing your activities in the way we described in earlier sections will make this happen less. It can also help if you can remind yourself that this is something that will pass when you have had a rest. What doctors refer to as clinical depression is something much more serious, for which you do need help. We talk about this in much more detail in Chapter 22.

Maintaining self-esteem

It is important to preserve and improve your sense of self-esteem. Giving yourself proper credit for any achievement, no matter how small, is a good idea. Setting yourself small, realistic targets can help to give you a valuable sense of achievement.

It is very easy to concentrate on what goes wrong. Paying as much or more attention to what you are getting right can help to redress the balance. Thinking well of yourself is important. If you only look at what you are getting wrong, you are likely to have a lower opinion of yourself than if you pay equal attention to what you are getting right. One way to identify what works for you might be to keep a journal for a few weeks in which you only record successful events and good times (see Appendix 2). Once you can see what they were and how you achieved them, you can plan to do more in the same way.

It can also help if you are able to come back to taking pride in your appearance (at least some of the time). A becoming though easily maintained hairstyle, using make-up, or shaving regularly, even if nobody else can see the results, buying a new item of clothing (mail order can be useful), will all have a good effect on your morale.

Old problems

Some of the problems that you had before you were ill can still be with you. You may even find that you have more time to notice them now you are ill. Old anger, old grief, difficulties with relationships, and so on can add to present distress. Sometimes just bringing them out into the open and talking about them to a friend or relative can help, but you may decide that you would benefit by some professional help. This could be something to discuss with your doctor, who is likely to be able to point you in the right direction.

Stress

Most people with CFS/ME find that stress makes them feel worse. Too much stress will hold back improvement. It is not possible to avoid stress altogether and trying to cut it out completely just does not work. However, you can work both on reducing some of the stress in your life and on managing the inevitable remainder to make it less distressing. The techniques of problem solving that we discuss in Chapter 24 will be helpful. Relaxation and calm breathing (Chapter 13) will reduce the physical effects of stress on your body. Some of the stress in your life may be the result of poor communication between you and the people around you. In Chapter 25 we describe how this could be improved.

You may need to look at what particular things cause you stress and to think a bit about why this is. Talking it over with someone you trust can often help you to identify what stresses you most and then to find better ways of dealing with it.

Worry

Becoming ill is bound to produce many problems and worries—such as how you are going to cope practically and financially, how long your illness will continue, and whether you are going to get worse—to add to any worries you already had. Managing worry, not letting it get out of hand, should be an important part of your strategy.

Limiting your worry

In Chapter 15 we talked about giving yourself a defined 'worry time'. What you need to avoid is thinking round and round your problems most of the time (which will be distressing, tiring, and inefficient). If you can restrict your thinking about problems to just one time each day, you are likely to be able to deal with them much more effectively. If a problem comes into your mind at another time, acknowledge it but tell yourself that you will think about it during your worry time. Some people find that it helps if they make a note of the problem, so that they can be confident that they will remember it and consider it later.

Keeping things in proportion

If you have many problems and worries, they can at times seem overwhelming. It is a common experience in illnesses of many kinds that people view problems in a different way than they did when they were well. Any problem can seem to be threatening. Talking things over with someone else can often enable you to get worries into proportion. With each difficulty, could you stand back a little and say to yourself: 'This is not a threat; it's just a problem. I'll deal with it now or later, but I won't go on thinking about it all the time.'?

Dealing with worry

You may decide to try the experiment of giving yourself a 'worry time', but how can you use it most effectively? It certainly will help if you are very structured in your approach. Separate out your worries, being specific about what they are, and then try to deal with them one at a time. The techniques of problem solving that we talk about in Chapter 24 will be useful in deciding what you can do about whatever is worrying you. Accept that some problems cannot be solved immediately; put that worry aside for the time being and concentrate on things that you can deal with now. Quite often you will find that a worry looked at calmly during the day seems much less important than when it filled your mind during the night. Try to keep a sense of proportion and check on the accuracy of your fears. Once you have given your worries an airing, move on to distracting yourself from them.

Distraction

Finding ways of distracting yourself can be very important. This usually means doing something else or thinking about something else, so that you can stop thinking about the worry for a while and give yourself a period of respite. Experiment with different distractions (doing something you enjoy or thinking about something else absorbing that will blot out the worry) and find out what works best for you.

Counselling

People with CFS/ME who have the problems with mood that we have described often believe that counselling will be of value to them, but have a rather vague idea of how or why. As counselling is often expensive and/or for a limited number of sessions, it is sensible to think carefully about what you want from it before you start. A definite goal such as 'I would like to deal better with such-and-such' will enable you to get the most value from the counselling sessions. If you can select one or two topics that distress you the most, you can work on these with the counsellor. If you get those resolved, you can always move on to something else.

Anything that you can do to improve your mood will have a positive effect on your body. Think about ways in which you could start managing your feelings of loss, frustration, anger, and fear. If old problems are still bothering you, this could be a time to get help with them. Getting better at dealing with stress and with worry will also help a lot. Counselling can sometimes be useful, particularly if you can define what help you want.

22
Managing anxiety, panic, and depression

Some people with CFS/ME also suffer from anxiety, panic, or depression, but many others do not. However, you are certainly not alone if you do experience this sort of thing. You may perhaps have had a tendency to this before you got ill or it may be a new and unwelcome burden. Anxiety and panic are very unpleasant to experience and produce physical symptoms which do not help your body, so anything you can do to control these emotional states will be of benefit to your general well-being. Feeling really anxious most of the time will certainly put added pressure on your body. Panic attacks can be exhausting, leaving you feeling really ill afterwards. Depression can cause physical symptoms and reduce your motivation, making managing your illness harder.

Anxiety

Real anxiety is different from just feeling a bit worried a lot of the time. For some people it can mean waking up in the morning in a state of total dread. They may not even be quite certain just what it is that is making them feel so anxious. Part of it is likely to be uncertainty about the future; part of it might be a feeling that their life is out of their control. Anything that can be done to identify the fears is likely to help. Bringing fears out into the open and then deciding what could be done if the worst happened can give you more sense of control. You may find that when you have identified your fears, you can see that some of them are excessive or exaggerated.

Physical symptoms

One of the added problems is that a state of anxiety can produce physical symptoms that are very similar to those of CFS/ME. This can then add extra worries about whether your illness is getting worse, which can increase your anxiety. Physical symptoms of anxiety can include:

palpitations, breathlessness, sweating, dry mouth, nausea, diarrhoea, twitching and shaking, muscle tension and fatigue. Fast, shallow breathing (hyperventilation) may be one of the things that adds to the physical symptoms.

What helps?

It will certainly help if you can reassure yourself that an increase in symptoms is due to your anxiety and that when you are less anxious they will subside. All the techniques of relaxation, calm breathing, and distraction that we talked about earlier will help. Talking things over with someone you trust is also a good idea. We give details in the reading list of books that will help you in anxiety management. Good research has shown that self-help techniques can be very effective.

Sometimes the level of anxiety is too great for self-help to be enough. Getting professional help may be necessary. Your doctor or therapist might suggest that you try one of the antidepressants that have been proved be effective in reducing anxiety. You will certainly be helping your body if you give this a try. We talk more about antidepressants later in this chapter. Tranquillizers are useful for a very short-term anxiety but are much better avoided long term. You may also benefit from a form of cognitive behaviour therapy specially tailored to dealing with anxiety. There is more about this in Chapter 32.

Panic

Some people with CFS/ME can have the extremely distressing experience of panic attacks—'an intense feeling of apprehension or impending doom, which is associated with a wide range of distressing physical sensations'. These attacks may be so severe that some people experiencing them fear that they are having a heart attack or that they will pass out. As many panic attacks are associated with the fear of something dreadful happening when away from home, some people can also develop agoraphobia (a fear of leaving the safety of the house) which can be distressingly restrictive.

What helps

Obviously panic attacks and the associated physical symptoms will add to the problems of CFS/ME, so learning how to manage and control them is important. One technique that may seem to help in the short term but actually makes things worse in the longer term is avoidance—avoiding the places or the circumstances in which panic attacks are likely to occur. Try not to avoid what you fear; instead try to manage the feelings of panic. There are techniques that have been proved to work.

It is always easier to deal with panic as it is starting, rather than when it has built up into a full-blown panic attack. If you can recognize the early-warning signs, you can start the techniques of relaxation and calm, slow breathing that will damp down the physical reactions. You can also look at some of your fears and check whether they are accurate. For example, is this chest pain really a heart attack?

If you have frequent panic attacks, do get help from your doctor or from someone trained to deal with such things. Both psychological treatment and anti-depressant drugs can cure panic. Help is available, so do ask for it.

Depression

Low mood some of the time is a normal reaction to having an illness such as CFS/ME. Many patients find that their mood goes down when they get exhausted, so pacing will help. Using the techniques we have discussed earlier to give your body a chance to improve will reduce your feelings of helplessness and hope-lessness. Getting better at dealing with your problems will give you a greater sense of control of your life. However, if you find yourself feeling really low for much of the time, it is very important that you should get help. If you find yourself thinking seriously about suicide, you really do need help. At this stage it is not that important whether your depression is a reaction to the difficulties caused by your illness or whether you were depressed before you became ill. Just recognize it as something that can be treated.

What is depression?

The symptom that most people associate with a 'depressive illness' is low mood, but there are many other symptoms as well. In fact, it is possible to suffer from depression without feeling depressed! The con-dition can show up as anxiety or extreme irritability. It can produce symptoms such as fatigue, pain, lack of energy or motivation, difficulty concentrating, reduced libido (sexual interest and drive), and lack of interest in food leading to weight loss. You may be thinking of some of your symptoms as due to CFS/ME, when they are actually caused by depression. It is not surprising that it can be difficult to differentiate between CFS/ME and depression.

Suffering depression does not mean that you are weak or pathetic. There is evidence that depression can have a physical basis (an imbalance of neurotrans-mitters in the brain). Unfortunately, there is still a social stigma about any illness that can be thought of as 'mental', though this is getting much less. Do try not to be ashamed of it. It can be tempting to think 'I'm not the sort of person to get depressed', but do you really know who does get depressed? Accept that it is an extra burden for you now, but one that can be treated. Be tolerant of family and friends if they find it easier to deny your depression.

Seasonal affective disorder

Some people with CFS/ME find that their mood and their symptoms get worse in the autumn and improve in the spring. It may be that they are suffering from what is called seasonal affective disorder (SAD). It is possible that seeing less sunlight during the winter months has an effect on parts of the brain. Some sufferers have found that regular use of a light box (sitting in front of a very bright light for several hours each day) can be helpful. However, it is a time-consuming and cumbersome remedy—taking a suitable antidepressant drug may be a more practical option.

Antidepressant drugs

Your doctor may suggest that you try an antidepressant. You might well have some concerns about taking such drugs. It could be helpful if we look more closely at some of these concerns:

- Some people simply dislike the idea of taking these drugs, feeling that they should be able to manage their problems themselves. This is an entirely understandable and laudable view, but although antidepressants will not change your problems, they are very likely to help you to a state in which you are better able to deal with them. You do not have to think in terms of drugs *or* self-help. You could use both.

- Others feel that their condition is not depression and therefore an antidepressant is not an appropriate drug. As we have said earlier in Chapter 6, the term 'antidepressant' is a misnomer. Rather than worry about the name, it may be better to use anything that works.

- Many people think that antidepressant drugs may be addictive or cause long-term harm. This is understandable, particularly given the reputation of the tranquillizing benzodiazepines, such as diazepam (Valium) for being addictive and producing very nasty withdrawal effects when stopped. This is a misconception. Some of the newer antidepressant drugs may cause some increase in symptoms if they are stopped suddenly, but these are not addictive drugs and you will not be able to sell them in your local night-club!

How to take an antidepressant

All drugs have some side-effects and antidepressants are no exception to this rule. Starting with a small dose and building up gradually will reduce the chance of such effects. This can be particularly important in a condition like CFS/ME in which many patients seem to be particularly sensitive to the side-effects of drugs. However, it is important in treating depression to work up to a full therapeutic dose (as recommended by your doctor) in order to see just how much help the drug may be. The danger of only trying it at a low dose is that you could end up rejecting something as ineffective which might have been very helpful at a higher dose.

One of the curious things about antidepressants is that they take a while to become effective. Although you may benefit almost immediately from a sedative effect, you are quite likely to notice side-effects before you feel other benefits. Most of these drugs do not start to have beneficial effects on energy and mood for at least two to four weeks after starting to take them at the therapeutic dose. Be prepared for a period during which you experience side-effects but not much benefit. There is a general agreement that a fair trial of these drugs is six weeks at full dose. Clearly, if the benefits do not outweigh the disadvantages at this stage it is a good idea to talk to your doctor about stopping the drug.

Although no major harm can come to you from stopping any of these drugs suddenly, it is generally wise to reduce the dose gradually. For some of the drugs that may cause brief withdrawal symptoms, this method will minimize the chance of this happening.

How to choose an antidepressant

Antidepressant drugs require a prescription. Your doctor will therefore guide you in which drug to take. An experienced doctor or a psychiatrist can select the antidepressant that is the most suitable for you. Some of the drugs have a sedative effect, which can be helpful if you are having problems with sleep. Others are somewhat energizing, which can be helpful if you have problems in getting going in the morning or in motivating yourself to action. Some drugs seem to have more effect on anxiety than others. There is no single antidepressant that works best for people with CFS/ME. It is very much a matter of 'horses for courses'.

The different types of antidepressant

There are four main types of antidepressants that are commonly used to treat depression, though other drugs are used as well.

The tricyclics

The advantage of these is that they have been used by millions of patients for over forty years, so a lot is known about them. They are known to be effective and we can be reasonably confident that they have no long-term harmful effects. The disadvantage is that they are toxic in overdose and they do tend to cause some degree of side-effects—the principal ones being a dry mouth, reduction in the ability of the eye to cope with bright lights at night, and sometimes a tremor. Other side-effects will be listed with the medicine. Many of these drugs are sedative, so taken at night they can aid sleep. Although the side-effects sound unpleasant, many people prefer these tried-and-tested drugs. Examples are amitriptyline (Tryptizol or Elavil), imipramine (Tofranil), and clomipramine (Anafranil). There are newer modifications of these, such as dothiepin (Prothiaden, not available in the USA), lofepramine (Gamanil, not available in the USA), and trazodone (Molipaxin or Desyrel).

The MAOIs

The monoamine oxidase inhibitors (MAOIs) are an old category of drugs that are now enjoying something of a revival. These drugs are potentially of interest for the treatment of CFS/ME as they seem to be particularly helpful for people afflicted by low energy, and those with a feeling of heaviness, 'leaden limbs', and increased sleep. The principal disadvantage of these drugs is that they work by affecting an enzyme in the body that occurs not only in the brain but also in the digestive system. This leads to people using these drugs being intolerant of a small range of food. The list of 'banned' foods includes those that contain a chemical called tyramine and includes certain red wines (especially Chianti), game, yeast extract, and some cheeses. Eating these foods can cause some quite severe reactions. As long as these foods are avoided, a normal diet is possible. The older MAOIs are phenelzine (Nardil) and tranylcypromine (Parnate). A more recent version is moclobemide (Manerix, not available in the USA). This has less stringent dietary requirements but many clinicians feel that it is not as effective as the older versions.

The SSRIs

The selective serotonin reuptake inhibitors (SSRIs) raise the level of the chemical serotonin (one of the neurotransmitters in the brain). They are as effective as the older drugs but are safer in overdose and have fewer side-effects. However, they may not be as effective in reducing pain. The principal side-effect is nausea. Common examples are fluoxetine (Prozac), sertraline (Lustral or Zoloft), citalopram (Cipramil or Celaxa), and fluvoxamine (Faverin or Fluvox).

The newer agents

Pharmaceutical companies are continually striving to develop more effective drugs that work rapidly and have fewer side-effects. The advantage of these is that they represent the pinnacle of pharmaceutical development, but the disadvantage is that we cannot yet be certain that there are no long-term effects. Examples of these drugs are venlafaxine (Efexor) and mirtazapine (Zispin or Remeron).

Multiple drugs

Doctors will sometimes give drugs in combination to people who do not respond to taking a single agent. This can sometimes be hazardous and so is usually only done on the advice of specialists. One potentially useful combination is a non-sedative drug in the morning and a sedative one at night. For example, many patients benefit from an SSRI, such as sertraline, taken in the morning and a sedative antidepressant drug, such as trazodone, taken at night. Such combinations should only be used under the supervision of a doctor.

Non-pharmaceutical antidepressants

People who dislike taking the products of the pharmaceutical industry for whatever reason sometimes ask if it is appropriate to take herbal preparations that are claimed to have an antidepressant action. One such preparation is 'St John's Wort' (*Hypericum perforatum*). There is evidence that this herb has an action similar to the antidepressants described above.

Some people do experience side-effects from it. It can conflict with some prescribed drugs, so you should always check with your doctor before taking it. This apparently 'natural' alternative does have a significant disadvantage. It can be very difficult to judge the quality and the quantity of what you are taking. Whatever one thinks about the pharmaceutical companies, they produce drugs of great purity in very carefully controlled doses. It is very much harder to do this with herbal preparations.

Non-drug alternatives

Some people with CFS/ME find that they are unable to tolerate the side-effects of antidepressants, even if they start them off very slowly. This does *not* mean that there is nothing that can be done to treat depression. There are other ways of tackling the problem. Cognitive behaviour therapy (CBT) was first developed as a treatment for depression, though it is now used for many other illnesses too. CBT for depression aims to help a patient look at the inaccurately negative thoughts and beliefs that are 'pushing mood down' and replacing them with more accurate ones. It is a collaborative process between a patient and a therapist. We talk more about CBT in Chapter 32. Many research trials have shown that it can be as effective a treatment as antidepressants. Although it is very much easier to do this with a trained therapist, it is possible to do a good deal of this by yourself. We recommend self-help books in the reading list.

Other things can help too. One of the things that can trigger depression is to find yourself in a very difficult, distressing situation over which you feel you have no control (which sounds very much like a description of CFS/ME if you do not know how to manage it). As you get better at managing your illness, you will get an increased sense that you are in control and that optimism about the future is possible. Research has shown that practising problem solving (see Chapter 24) can help with depression. Finding someone who will listen to you is always helpful, particularly if they understand about depression. You really can believe that this black patch will pass and that you will come out the other side.

Anything you can do to improve your mood and to cope better with anxiety, panic, and depression will be of real benefit to your body as well as making your life easier. You could read some of the self-help books we recommend and practise the techniques they suggest. Depression is something that can and should be treated. It is not a sign of weakness. You do not need to feel ashamed of depression or hesitate in asking for help.

23
Managing your thinking

Understanding the way you think—the way you view yourself, your life, and the world around you—can make a great difference to the way you manage your illness. We all of us, well or ill, have established patterns in the way we think. Some of these are helpful and some unhelpful, but they all influence our feelings and our mood. Moods and emotions have a physical effect on the body, which is why we believe that managing your thinking is so important. Some of your beliefs and thought patterns may well have been appropriate in the past but no longer fit the person you are today.

We can point out some specific ways of thinking that are common in a lot of people and mention how they can get in the way of good management of CFS/ME, but you are going to be the best person to judge just how much any of them apply to you. We are *not* saying that the only reason you are still ill is because of the way you think. What we *are* saying is that changing some unhelpful thought patterns may make life better for you and make it easier for you to stick to your self-help programme.

Thinking that the worst is likely to happen

You may have got into the habit of always expecting the worst, of believing that if anything can go wrong for you it will do so. This can make things a lot more difficult if you have CFS/ME. You are likely to fear that any new symptom means that your illness is deteriorating or even that it is a sign of a life-threatening condition. If you expect things to turn out badly, you are likely to be hesitant at trying anything new.

Black-and-white thinking

In this style of thinking everything is either good or bad, helpful or unhelpful, perfect or a disaster. If you stick to just black or white, you can miss out on the interesting shades of grey in between. You are likely to consider that you are either perfectly well or hopelessly ill, when the realistic viewpoint might be that you are considerably improved, but not yet in perfect health. Things are either catastrophes or successes instead of a mixed bag of a bit of failure and a bit of success. You are likely to believe that if you do not do something perfectly you have failed, instead of thinking (accurately) that you did pretty well in the circumstances.

Negative thinking

This is very common, particularly if you are feeling a bit depressed. You are likely to always believe the worst, particularly about yourself and the way people are reacting to you. Typical thoughts could be:

- 'I'm a failure'
- 'I always get things wrong'
- 'Everybody dislikes me'
- 'I'm never going to get better'.

If you look again at those last three thoughts, you will notice that they contain very absolutist words like 'always', 'everybody', and 'never'. This is very typical of negative thinking, when other words like 'sometimes' and 'some people' would be much more accurate and 'never' could be replaced by a concept like 'it may take a long time'. Identifying and challenging these negative thoughts and looking at alternative, more accurate ones can make things seem much better.

Mind-reading

This is a very common problem. You presume that you know what people are thinking about you and it is usually rather negative. 'They think I'm not trying hard enough.' 'They don't believe that I really am ill.' That *might* be true, but it probably is not. Checking up on the accuracy of your beliefs is always worthwhile.

Believing that if a thing happened once, it will happen again

This covers things like believing that if you failed once, it means that you will always go on failing. It can be important to challenge this, particularly when it comes to managing your illness and pacing. A typical thought would be: 'I tried pacing myself last week and it didn't work. There is no point trying again.'

The 'socially acceptable' model

Another important area to consider is your own model of what makes you a 'good person'. In a society that is very much concerned with achievement, you may well feel devalued by being able to do much less. If you have had to give up your job, your own sense of worth may have sunk. The 'model' you had before you were ill may have suited you then (though it might have been one of the things that made you more vulnerable to CFS/ME) but it may be totally inappropriate to your state now. It can be very helpful to look at your own ideas and judge whether they are helpful or unhelpful. The 'good person' model can often lead to you believing that you ought to be doing more than is appropriate or worrying that you are not doing enough. Our impression is that women tend to be more susceptible to pressures in this way, often believing that they ought to give their own needs a lower priority than those of their families or of those around them.

Guilt

Another thing that comes up a lot in chronic illness (not just in CFS/ME) is guilt. So many of the people we talk with feel guilty about some aspect of their illness. This is often tied up with the concept of 'blame'. You may find it helpful to consider whether you would blame someone else in your position. It can sometimes be very difficult to convince people with CFS/ME that when we suggest ways in which they could manage their illness better that we are not blaming them for being ill, which we certainly are not. Some people tend to assume that if you become ill and stay ill it is somehow your fault. For people suffering from CFS/ME this may be made worse by the suggestion that they are really just lazy. These comments are ignorant and unfair and can make managing illness so much more difficult. Try to ignore them.

Challenging unhelpful thinking

So what if you have decided that some of your thought patterns are unhelpful? What can you do about it? There are some well-tried and tested methods of challenging inappropriate and outdated thinking. Mostly they consist of asking yourself questions like:

- 'What is the evidence that supports this belief?'
- 'Would I apply these standards to somebody else I cared about?'

You can get better at recognizing unhelpful thinking and then challenging it—along the lines of:

- 'OK, that is one way of thinking, that is one interpretation of events. Are there any others?'
- 'What could I do to gather evidence to judge whether this thought is accurate?'

We talk about this in more detail in Chapter 32 and we give details in the reading list of some books that you could find helpful.

Other things to consider

There are some other ways of thinking about yourself and your illness that can help or hinder your improvement.

Aiming for normality

However severe your condition, there is more to your life than your illness. You are still a person of worth, even though you are ill, and you can contribute to life and take an interest in things other than illness. You do not have to think of yourself as *only* a person with CFS/ME. The more you concentrate on your illness and the difficulties of your life now, the worse you are likely to feel. 'Symptom scanning' is likely to make you notice symptoms much more and mind about them much more. Thinking and behaving in as normal a way as possible in the circumstances is going to make your life better. You need to balance pacing and sensible behaviour with the need to be 'ordinary'.

Balancing acceptance and hope

So many people with CFS/ME who have got a lot better tell us that they can look back and see that real improvement started when they *accepted* what was happening to them. 'This is not what I wanted. I do not have to like it, but it is what is happening today. How can I make the most of my material?' This kind of acceptance does not mean that you have to give up hope for future improvement, rather the reverse. It is only when you are accurate in your thinking about today that you can start working on an improved tomorrow and so be more optimistic about the future.

> Unhelpful and inaccurate thinking can make your life much more difficult now that you are ill and can get in the way of managing your illness. Recognizing and challenging your unhelpful or inaccurate thoughts and beliefs can be a very useful step towards recovery.

24
Dealing with problems

We all face difficulties and problems in our lives. However, being ill can create a new batch of problems to go with the ones you had before. At every stage of your illness things change; some problems get easier, but new ones crop up—even getting better can cause some problems! Managing problems in the best way is very much part of managing your illness and giving yourself the best chance of improvement.

Before going on to consider how best to deal with problems, you might like to think about the difference between difficult circumstances and problems. Many of the people we talk to seem to be trying to solve the difficult circumstances, rather than dealing with the problems that those circumstances produce.

As we said earlier, when you are feeling ill and tired, problems seem to loom larger. It is very likely that you will have times when *any* problem can seem very threatening. If you have lots of them, it can seem almost impossible to know where to start and how to find any solutions. Nevertheless, if you can hang on to the idea that they are just problems, not threats, you can do more about finding solutions. With each problem that you solve, you will get better at dealing with others and you will build up confidence in your own abilities.

Problem solving

One of the life skills that will be particularly useful to you now is called 'problem solving'. There has been a lot of research into this subject to find what works best. What follows is just a summary of the technique; in the reading list at the end of the book we point you to books you can read that will give you more guidance. What we suggest is that you start with just one fairly simple problem. You can then tackle it in seven stages:

Stage 1: Identifying and clarifying the problem

It is going to be much easier to tackle any problem if you can identify exactly what it is and separate it out from all the rest of the stuff that is bothering you.

1. What exactly is the problem?
2. When and where does the problem occur?
3. What other people does it involve?

Be very specific; do not muddle it up with others. Give it a name. Write down a clear description of the problem.

John had been ill for three years and was not well enough to work. He lived on his own, though he had a brother living nearby. He knew that he was letting his paperwork get out of hand. There were bills, official forms, and letters strewn around in a complete muddle, so that he spent a lot of time looking for a specific bit of paper and was often late paying bills. This worried him, but the whole thing seemed such a mess that he kept putting off dealing with it.

Stage 2: Deciding on your goal or goals

Set yourself a goal of what would change things for the better, rather than a somewhat vague hope for improvement. Choose a goal that you know you can achieve and make it very definite.

John realized that he had two goals associated with this problem: to get his paperwork into order and to clear up the backlog of unanswered mail. He decided to tackle the sorting out first.

Stage 3: Thinking of as many solutions as possible

'Brainstorming' can be a useful technique. It is a good idea to use a pencil and paper at this stage. Your aim is to identify as many solutions as possible, writing each one down, and not stopping to think about whether any of them would work until you have run out of ideas. Having someone you trust doing this with you can be useful as they might be able to suggest ideas you might not have thought about. You do not need to reject *any* idea at this stage, even if it seems to be ridiculous. Do not stop and say 'Oh but that wouldn't work.' Only when you have got your complete list in front of you should you start to evaluate the solutions. Ask yourself what are the pros and cons of each one.

John asked his brother to help him with the brainstorming. Together they made up a list of solutions that included paying someone else to sort things out, letting his brother do it for him, doing all of it himself right away, doing it himself but in smaller bites, and buying some coloured files.

Stage 4: Choosing the best solution and deciding how to put it into practice

When you have got your list of solutions in front of you and have thought about each one, you can choose the best solution. That is the one that seems to be the most practical and which fits your situation best.

John decided that he would prefer to do the sorting out himself, but not all at once which would be too tiring. He decided to set aside twenty minutes each day to sort papers. He would get his brother to buy him some coloured files to put them in when they were sorted.

When you feel happy about the solution, break it down into steps. 'I could begin by doing this and then move on to doing that.' Be very definite about what you are going to do and when you are going to do it.

John decided that his steps would be:
  to go round gathering up all the papers and to put them on the dining table;
  to sort them all out into piles—bills, official forms, letters to be answered, urgent, etc.;
  to label the files;
  to put each group of papers into the appropriate file in date order.
He would make sure that he did at least twenty minutes every day, though if he felt up to it he would come back to the task later in the day.

Stage 5: Trying it out

There is no point in having a potential solution if you do not use it. If you start finding good reasons *not* to try out the solution, it probably was not the right one, or you may have chosen too big a problem to begin with and would perhaps do better to tackle just part of the problem.

Once John got going, he found that it only took him a week to get everything sorted. Having got things in order, he could see what needed doing urgently and what could wait.

Stage 6: Evaluating the success of the solution

When you have put the solution into practice, check on whether it is working. It can be helpful to discuss this with someone. You will have learned a lot from any mistakes you have made.

Though John had got things sorted out, it still took him some time to catch up on the backlog of things he had not done, which worried him a little. He thought that it might have been better to have accepted some help from his brother. However, he felt that he could now start to work out a system that would keep things in order.

Stage 7: Beginning again

If the problem is solved, congratulate yourself. If not, start again at step one and decide if it was the best problem to tackle. If you still think it was, try an alternative solution and progress through the stages as last time. You can then go on to tackle other problems in the same way.

Do keep in mind that some problems do not have obvious solutions or cannot be tackled yet, because you do not have enough information. Part of your technique for dealing with problems should be to accept that some things may have to be tolerated for the time being. Another important part may be to accept that you may have to postpone doing any work on some problems until you have gathered more information. You cannot make realistic decisions without enough data.

Life is full of difficulties and problems, but getting better at dealing with them in a structured way will reduce stress and make you feel more in control of your life:

- identify the problem
- decide on your goal
- think of as many solutions as possible
- choose the best solution and decide how to put it into practice
- try it out
- evaluate its success
- if that solution did not work, go back and try another solution. If it did work, move on to another problem.

Accept that some problems cannot be solved just now.

25
Better communications

One of the things that can add to the difficulty of managing any long-term illness is poor communications between you and the people around you—family, friends, doctors, officials, employers, etc. Getting a message across clearly and calmly can do a lot to make a difficult situation easier and reduce stress, so it should definitely be part of your plan for helping yourself. Good communication is a skill that can be improved with practice.

These are some topics that we think are particularly relevant to your present situation.

Quiet assertiveness

You will communicate better if you can be quietly assertive, but that is easier to do if you believe that you still have rights. It is all too easy to slip into the trap of believing that you have stopped having rights since becoming ill. It can be very helpful to think about your own rights, taking your illness into account. You could try thinking about the rights you would give to somebody else in your circumstances such as:

- the right to look after themselves and not be pushed into doing something that would tire them too much
- the right to say 'no'
- the right to choose what help they accept
- the right to use some of their energy for pleasure.

Balance your rights against the rights of the people around you. It is a two-way process. Other people have rights that need to be thought about.

Once you have a list of your own rights that feels comfortable to you, you will be in a much better position to be quietly assertive about what you want and what you need.

Explaining an invisible illness

It is very natural that you should want the people around you to understand what is happening to you and their lack of understanding can be a cause of friction and distress. CFS/ME can be an invisible illness. Fatigue, malaise, and pain may not show. Often people only see you when you are well enough to get out or to see visitors, so they tend to judge you by how you appear then. Although more people are learning about CFS/ME, there is no reason why they *ought* to understand unless they are given the facts. (Did you know much about it before you became ill?) It is always worth checking up on what other people do or do not know and then filling in the gaps. Do not expect them to understand what you have not told them. You have a right to choose whether or not to tell some people about your CFS/ME, but you have to accept that if you do not tell them, they may think of you as a well person.

Sufferers often want *all* the people around them to understand *all* about the illness, but it can be worth thinking about this in a more specific way. Try thinking about one particular person. What do you feel that you are not getting from that person because of their lack of understanding? Then ask yourself these questions:

1. What particular aspect of your illness do you want them to understand?

2. What information would help them to understand?

3. What would they be saying or doing that would show that they did understand?

4. Is what you want something they can give?

5. Is it reasonable to expect them to give it to you?

Once you have got that clear in your mind, you can start thinking about what information to give them and how to explain your reasonable needs. It may take time for them to adjust to this approach.

Asking for help

Many people find it difficult to ask for help. Some feel that they *ought* to be able to cope on their own and that it is a sign of weakness if they do not. Some fear rejection: 'What if they said no!' It is worth looking at your own feelings about this. A good working motto is 'I can ask anyone for anything as long as I respect their right to say no.'

Saying no yourself

You may find it very hard to refuse when you are asked to do something for or with someone else (although it should be on your 'rights' list to refuse if it would be too tiring or interfere with your pacing programme). One approach that can sometimes help is to turn down the whole request with a show of regret, but to offer something much smaller instead.

Practical suggestions

These are some suggestions for better communication that have been proved to help:

- Try to stay calm. There is something about strong emotion that makes people discount much of what you say. This is particularly true when talking to young people; emotion in a parent seems to produce selective deafness in teenagers! Anger certainly gets in the way.

- Keep it short and simple. Long-winded explanations often make people lose interest.

- If possible, tap into the experience of the people you are talking to. For instance, if you are trying to explain the overwhelming exhaustion you may experience, try reminding them of a time when they experienced something similar (like reminding a mother what it was like when she had a teething baby keeping her awake at night as well as an active toddler). When you have pointed out what is similar, you can outline the differences—for example, it may not take much to get you exhausted and a 'good night's sleep' probably will not make you feel much better.

- Try to stand back sometimes and look at things from the other person's point of view. If you feel that you have good cause to complain about what they are doing (or not doing) try to stick to criticisms of their actions, not of them as people.

- Do your best to stay consistent, even though your condition may fluctuate. Try not to turn down help crossly one day when you are feeling a bit better and then be wounded another time because help is not offered.

- If someone asks you how you are, it is better not to answer 'Fine' automatically. If you usually say you are fine, people will assume that that is how you are. On the other hand, saying too much about how terrible you are feeling can make some people switch off. Try to find a balance between the two approaches.

- Give them something to read. This book might be a start!

If you have a specific point you want to get across, you will probably do better to write down in advance what you need to say, particularly if you have problems with memory and concentration. This can be a great help when you are talking to doctors or officials. You can then be sure that you have covered all the necessary points. Show that you appreciate that their time may be limited and keep it as brief as you can without missing out on anything important.

Clear, calm communications will reduce stress and save energy. If that is something you find difficult, read about it and practise your skills. The more you work at it, the easier it will become.

26

Managing relationships and people

Being ill often changes relationships. Even the best relationships can be put under strain and one that was a little rocky to begin with may become very difficult. You may be grieving for the past, for your lost job perhaps, or the things that you cannot do now. However, your illness may have affected others. A carer may have had to take on the responsibility of housework or earning the money and have had to give up a lot of things they enjoyed previously on their own or with you. Their grief needs to be acknowledged too. You may feel that they are not caring enough; they may feel that you are asking too much. There may be a lot of resentment on both sides.

A difficult relationship is an obvious cause of stress, which will not be helpful to you in your plan for improvement, so anything you can do to ease the relationship will be of benefit. There are no absolute rules, each person and each relationship is unique but some general guidelines might be:

- Keep communications open. Avoid 'mind-reading' (assuming that you know what the other person is thinking in a given situation). You could well be inaccurate in your assumptions.

- Check that the other person in the relationship knows the facts about your illness. Find simple ways of explaining how it affects you.

- If something in the relationship is bothering you, choose a time when you are both at your best to discuss the problem. Some people find that it helps to have a definite time once a week to talk over problems, with both sides having equal time to put their side of the picture.

- Spend a little time imagining yourself in their place and thinking about things from their point of view. This can often let you see that they are not being totally unreasonable.

- Accept that some people are not going to understand what your illness is like for you. With some friends or relations you may have to choose between going on seeing them, in spite of their lack of understanding, and cutting out that relationship for the time being. Some people do feel very uneasy about illness (it reminds them of their own potential vulnerability).

- In general, try to aim for negotiation rather than confrontation.

Bertha was very distressed and angry that her family were still expecting her to do all the housework in spite of her illness. After a while she realized that just moaning at them was not getting her anywhere. Instead, she chose a time when all of them were at their best and set up a family conference. She itemized all the things that needed doing and explained why she really was not capable of doing them all. She asked them to make suggestions as to which tasks each individual would prefer to do (rather than giving them orders) and then negotiated towards a solution that they all felt was fair.

- If relationships get very difficult and strained, it may be a good idea to seek professional help—family therapy or couple therapy for instance. Your doctor will probably be able to make suggestions as to how you could find this help.

Sexual relationships

If you have a partner, one of the areas that can cause difficulties and stress is that of your sexual relationship. If you are very tired or in pain, sex can be the last thing on your mind. Nevertheless, it is an important factor in your relationship. You may need to educate your partner so that he or she can consider positions and methods that are easier for the one with CFS/ME and also to think about different timing. Would mornings or afternoons be a better time for you than last thing at night? Do believe that sex does not necessarily have to be just about passion; warmth and affection, closeness and cuddling can be just as important. Sex can be energizing as well as exhausting.

Improving your relationship with your doctor

If you have an illness that is not going to improve quickly, having a good relationship with your doctor can make a great deal of difference. Even if it is not very good at the moment, it may be possible to improve it.

Sometimes people with CFS/ME expect too much from their doctors. It can be helpful to distinguish between what you *need* from doctors and what you *want* from them—you *need* appropriate medical treatment (which is what they were trained to do); you may *want* a degree of emotional support (which they may feel is not their role).

Once you are clear in your mind about what you need from your doctor, it can be very helpful to look at things from his or her point of view. Doctors these days have been trained to make diagnostic tests and then apply a treatment based on the results of those tests, so a condition like CFS/ME can be difficult for them.

These are suggestions about getting on better with doctors, based on what they have told us and what people with CFS/ME have told us:

- Doctors are often unhappy about the names ME or CFIDS for the condition as they feel they are technically inaccurate. It is probably more tactful to use the term CFS when talking to them (whatever you may call it to yourself).

- Doctors often dislike patients doing too much self-diagnosis (after all, it is what *they* were trained to do). It is generally better not to say 'I am sure I have got ME', but rather to describe your symptoms and then say something more indirect such as 'It has been suggested that I might have something like CFS.'

- Try to understand things from the doctor's point of view. Doctors like to make people feel better. CFS/

ME can be frustrating for them too. They work by looking for things that they *can* treat. That is why they may look hard for depression.

- Try not to be angry if your doctor suggests that you might be suffering from depression. The symptoms of depression can be quite similar to those of CFS/ME. Your illness may have features of both CFS/ME and depression. Doctors know that they can suggest treatment for depression.

- Show that you realize that your doctor's time is limited. Write down the points you want to cover and the questions you want to ask so that you can express yourself clearly and briefly. If there is a great deal to discuss, consider asking for a double appointment.

- Do not expect your doctor to feel the same about alternative therapies as you do. He or she may be comfortable with some but dismiss the rest.

- Many people with CFS/ME only see their doctor when they are well enough to get to the surgery or office. Keep your doctor informed about what it is like at the bad times.

- Being a patient with a chronic illness can be quite different from the days when you just visited a doctor for something specific like a sore throat. You may be able to discuss this new relationship with your doctor and together work out a new 'contract'.

- If you cannot get to the doctor, or have trouble choosing the right words when you do, try writing him or her a brief letter explaining the problem and saying what you want.

Your relationship with your doctor is an important one, so anything you can do to improve the partnership between the two of you will be of real benefit.

> Trying to improve relationships may be hard work, but it will certainly be of benefit to you. Remember that any relationship is a two-way process, so try to consider their side as well as your own. Being clear in the way you communicate is very important.

27
Getting the best from today

We hope that by trying out some of the strategies for self-help that we have outlined in previous chapters, your condition will start to improve (even if only very slowly) so that you can look forward to a better tomorrow.

But what about today? Improving the quality of your life today is something worth aiming for. You are bound to have times when you are frightened that you are never going to get any better and that what you are today is all you will ever be. It may be an exaggerated fear, but it can still be there. Making today better can reduce fears about tomorrow. These are some practical suggestions about how to improve today.

Making the most of a limited energy budget

At this stage you may well have to accept that the amount you can do is limited, so it is worth thinking about whether everything you are doing is essential or pleasurable. Some people find it helpful to think in terms of budgeting their energy expenditure in the same way they would budget a low income. You may have to make choices about whether you can afford something, whether it is in energy or money.

You could also think about whether you are 'spending' your energy efficiently. Using the same amount of energy to achieve a bit more is often possible if you think about it in a rather structured way. A good place to start is by considering your activities, mental as well as physical, under the headings of What?, Why?, How?, and When?

- What—could you reduce some of the things you do now by concentrating on essentials?
- Why—could you look at the reasons why you are doing what you do? Could it be because you have always done such-and-such, even though that is not really appropriate for you today?
- How—could you do the essentials in a more labour-saving way?
- When—could you spread your activities out during the day and during the week?

Changing the way in which you do things

If you are still doing things in the same way as you did before you were ill, you are likely to hit against obstacles and deny yourself possible pleasures or satisfactions. You may need to change your style quite a bit. One of the techniques that will help is to do a lot of forward planning, spreading out the task, and pacing yourself carefully. Being too perfectionist will certainly get in the way.

Clare used to enjoy having friends round for a meal and had very high standards when she entertained. After a few bad experiences, trying to do things in the same old style, she realized that her friends did not expect her to do so much. She thought about very simple food that could be prepared well in advance—something like a casserole and a cold pudding—and got almost everything ready the previous day. To her delight she found that the social occasion was just as successful as before and yet it did not exhaust her.

With anything that you would like to do but that seems beyond you at the moment, think carefully about whether it would be possible if you spread out the preparations in the previous day or days and kept things simple.

Equipment

You may decide that there are various pieces of equipment that would make your life easier or allow you to do more with your available energy. Before you invest in anything expensive, though, it can be worth asking yourself whether it is something you would use if you got a bit better. Obviously, something like a microwave cooker or a deep-freeze could be useful whatever your state of health. It is better not to rush into getting 'invalid aids' unless you really need them.

There may be small or inexpensive things that would make your life easier—even a more efficient can-opener could be helpful.

Building pleasure into your life today

If you are feeling tired and ill it can be hard to think about enjoying yourself. You may have a Puritanical feeling that you do not deserve pleasure while you are ill or you may feel that people will criticize you for using some of your available energy on things other than the essentials. However, pleasure is an essential part of your diet—just as important as good food. Often the things that used to give you pleasure are not possible at present, but that does not mean that you could not enjoy yourself in rather different ways. Now could be the time to try something a bit different.

You could try making a list of all the things you can think of that might give you pleasure or satisfaction, within the limits of your present condition. Keep it by you and add to it every time a new idea occurs to you. You might be surprised by how long a list you end up with.

Most people have things that they have always wanted to do but never had the time to try. This could be your time to do just a little of them.

Frankie had always had a fantasy about doing exquisite needlepoint embroidery, though she never found the right moment to learn the techniques. When she had been ill for a year, she realized that now was her chance. She bought a simple kit, which she did not do very well, but she learned from her mistakes and now does small amounts that give her real pleasure and satisfaction.

This could also be a time for you to learn more about subjects that have always interested you. Education does not just have to be about vocational training; it can be satisfying in its own right.

Many people with CFS/ME find that this is a time to explore their creative side—art, writing, and so on.

You know best what you might enjoy. Experiment, always remembering that fun is possible and that it will do you a lot of good. You really do have the right to enjoy yourself and indulge yourself.

Treats and rewards

One way of looking at things could be to imagine what you would do for friends in similar circumstances. You might buy flowers for them, pick out an amusing book, choose a nice video, get some food that you know they enjoy. Have you considered indulging yourself in this way? Why not give yourself these sorts of little treats, if only as a reward for the way you are coping with your illness?

Keeping in contact with the outside world

Unfortunately, being ill can mean that you lose out on a lot of the social activity you enjoyed before. Feeling isolated can be a very common problem for people with CFS/ME. Social contact is a basic human need and very necessary for you now. You may have to think about being social in a different way, like having a friend join you for a take-away meal instead of inviting several people round for a meal you prepared yourself.

You may also need to replace the friends who dropped away because they could not cope with you being ill. Making new social contacts can often seem difficult, but usually there are ways round the problem. There may be a CFS/ME support group in your area that you could join and meet people with similar problems, although these groups do vary enormously and you may find that your local one is not your style. If you cannot get out easily there may be local organizations that do home visits (perhaps one of the churches near you).

Socializing does not have to happen face to face. Pen-friends (a postcard, even if you cannot manage a letter) and telephone contacts can be very helpful. A lot of people with CFS/ME find that telephone calls are a lot less tiring anyway. You could also try e-mail. Anything you can do to keep in contact with the world is going to be good for you.

Improving the quality of your life today is very important, both in making life easier and in reducing fear and frustration. It can help if you look at all aspects of your life and think hard about small ways of making things a little better.

28
Managing employment

You may still be working (even with great difficulty) or you may have made enough improvement to be able to think about getting back to work. What would be the best way of managing employment without putting too much strain on yourself? As we have said before, each person and each situation is different, so there are no hard and fast rules. However, we can offer some general, tried-and-tested suggestions.

First of all, it can be a great help if your employer, your immediate superior, and your colleagues know about your illness and understand what it involves. However, this is not always desirable or possible. In some situations it may have an adverse affect on career prospects to have it known that you have a health problem; some employers may be reluctant to take on a new employee with a record of ill-health. You will have to be the best judge of this, but if you can be open about it, it will certainly make things easier.

You may have to accept that for a while you will have to limit what you do in the evenings and at weekends and concentrate your energies on the working day. Pacing yourself while you are at work is very important. Try to give yourself pauses during which you switch off and relax.

Everything we have said earlier about stress and stress management is particularly relevant in a working environment. It is worth giving a good deal of thought as to how you could reduce stress. Maybe you could go for a less demanding job; maybe you could get better at saying 'no' when unreasonable demands are made of you.

Communication and negotiation skills will certainly make your life easier. If the people around you do not understand about the limitations imposed on you by your condition, they may be resentful that you do not seem to be 'pulling your weight', which would add to your problems.

One of the books in our reading list will give you more ideas about how to manage your working life.

If you are still managing to hold down a job or if you are planning to return to work, then pacing, stress management, good communications, and problem solving will all help.

29

Thinking about the future

You may feel so stuck in your present problems that it is hard to envisage a better future, but the possibility is certainly there. As your health improves you will begin to see things opening up, some of which may seem pretty scary. If you have been ill for some time, getting back into the world, perhaps coming off benefits, and going back to work can seem very daunting. There are likely to be problems about being better, just as there have been problems about being ill. The more you can be clear about what the problems might be and what you might be able to do about them, the less scary it will be.

Getting back to work

When you reach the stage at which you can see the possibility of working again, you will need to think about whether you want to return to your old job. If you do, it will obviously be easier if you have kept in touch with your previous employer and can negotiate a gradual return—perhaps part-time to begin with or in a less-demanding role.

You may recognize that your previous occupation is no longer attractive to you. It could be that the stress involved in your previous job was one of the factors that made you vulnerable to illness. Your previous job may no longer be open to you. This could be a good time to review what you want to do in life. One technique that many people find helpful is to think hard about their previous job and analyse which bits were stressful, which bits were bearable (though perhaps boring), and which bits they really enjoyed. Once you have identified what aspects of your work gave you the most satisfaction, you may be able to see a new direction that would include more of that sort of thing.

It may be that you now feel that you really do not want to return to your previous career. At this stage, all you may be certain of is that you do not want to go back to what you used to do, but have no clear idea of what else might suit you. This could be a good time to consider a wide range of other possibilities, without committing yourself to anything. Your period of convalescence provides you with an opportunity to 'play' with things before committing yourself. As all you are doing is thinking about it, you do not need to limit your ideas. 'Do I fancy being an astronaut? Well perhaps not.' Maybe what would suit you is something similar to what you used to do; maybe you feel that you need a complete change of direction. Think hard about your strengths as well as your weaknesses. Gather as much information as possible to help you in your decision making. Your local library will have books about career choices. You may be able to get some kind of career guidance. You could talk to people who are already working in an area that interests you. You could certainly use the problem-solving techniques we discussed in Chapter 24.

Voluntary and part-time work

Quite often, the way back into employment can be through some kind of voluntary work, even if it is only for an hour or two per week. Just getting back into the world and doing something can be of benefit, but it could be even better if it is in an area that interests you. That way you could get a taste of that sort of thing.

Voluntary work has other benefits. Many people find that they have lost confidence while they have been ill. Working with other people, even if you are not getting paid for it, can be one way of rebuilding that confidence. It can also be helpful to be able to say to a prospective employer that you have been doing something like this.

You may well be able to do a part-time job for a while without losing out on any benefits. Part of your information gathering may require talking to the officials administering your benefit to find out just how many hours you would be allowed to do or how much you would be allowed to earn without affecting your benefit. Later on, when you feel able to work longer hours, you could also investigate government schemes to help people with disabilities get back to work. If you are at present receiving Permanent Health Insurance income, you could find out from the insurance company whether they allow part-time working while still getting some benefit.

Both voluntary and part-time work can be routes back to normal living.

Education

Part of your plan for dealing with improvement might include education for a new career. You could start this in a very modest way, perhaps by just getting one book about a possible new direction and reading it slowly. Later on you may decide on retraining, but again this can be done modestly—one class a week to begin with and then an increase later on when you feel up to it.

Managing a relapse

Even if you seem to be improving steadily, there are likely to be times when you slip back a bit. Maybe feeling better will tempt you into doing a little too much, too quickly; maybe you will pick up an infection; maybe you will meet with an unexpected stress. Whatever the cause for a relapse, it could feel extremely frightening. You may tend to think in catastrophic terms: 'I'm going back to where I was. I'm never going to get better again.' Of course that is not true. You will have just had a set-back and can deal with it. Your forward planning needs to include thinking about how you would deal with a relapse. If you can think of a relapse as just a minor set-back that can be managed as you have managed before, it will be much less frightening.

Managing change

We have talked about getting back to work, but there will probably be other areas in which you will have to adapt to a changed role as someone well rather than someone ill. You may have to move back to taking responsibility for things that you handed over to others while you were ill. You may need to work slowly at rebuilding your confidence at doing things on your own. You may need to think in terms of rehabilitation—like getting used to driving again, perhaps with someone with you to start with and then short trips on your own. Doing things gently and not rushing into complete independence will probably make it easier.

While you were ill you might have had very little chance of meeting new people and have lost confidence in your social skills. Getting back to it can be difficult. Some people find that it helps if they deliberately seek out opportunities to meet people in a non-stressful way.

Martin decided that one way to get back to socializing again would be to join a local weekly photography class. He would be likely to meet people there with similar interests. He was very nervous the first week, but found that it got easier. He enjoyed the class and made a couple of friends.

It is a fact of life, though one that may come as something of an unpleasant surprise, that not everyone will necessarily welcome your re-emergence into normal living. Some of the people around you may have got used to you being ill and actually enjoyed having you dependent on them. Because they found a role for themselves in being carers, they may now feel somewhat challenged by your increasing independence. Some relationships that worked well while you were ill may crumble once you become better, but some may just need to be renegotiated.

Sam's partner was very supportive while he was ill. When he started getting better and began to do things for himself, he realized that she was not totally happy for him. She had obviously got something from being the person who did things for him and supported him. His independence was something of a threat. They had to work together at redefining their changed relationship.

A new way of looking at life

It is possible that the pace of your life before you were ill was not sensible and was more than you could have kept up indefinitely. You might have been burning the candle at both ends. If this was the case it would probably be unwise to go back to that sort of lifestyle. Part of your planning for the future should include thinking about why you pushed yourself so hard and accepting that repeating this pattern of behaviour would be a mistake. You may have to give up some ambitions and recognize that some of your previous activities are no longer possible. Pacing yourself more carefully to limit excessive demands may have to be part of your life for some time to come. The style of managing yourself that we have talked about is likely to give you a real improvement, but it is not a guaranteed cure. You may need to be careful for a long time, but you do not have to think of this as second-best. Being gentle with yourself could well be a life skill that will be of real benefit to you for the rest of your life.

It is possible to use this period in a constructive way. You have time to think about what you liked and did not like in your life before you were ill and, based on that, plan out a better future.

Getting better can be wonderful, but it can also pose a challenge. Accepting that there are problems can be the first stage in dealing with them. Lots of forward planning and information gathering will help. Voluntary or part-time work may be the route back into full employment. Relationships may have to be redefined. You may need to plan for a very different lifestyle from the one you had before you were ill, but different does not have to be worse.

30
Summary of our self-help advice

We very much hope that you will try out the self-help techniques that we have outlined in this section. Research and clinical experience have shown that they *can* result in an improvement in your condition. Over time they can make a great difference to your state of health and to your well-being. In the ten years and more that we have been working with people with CFS/ME, we have seen the benefits that can come from this approach. We do not say that these techniques will give you a cure, but they can give you the significant benefits of a decrease in symptoms and/or an increase in your level of functioning. You could try to:

- stabilize your rest/activity pattern, work towards improving your sleep, see that you eat healthily, learn to relax and to manage pain. Aim for consistency;

- manage your difficulties with memory and concentration;

- do your best to behave as normally as possible;
- start the process of making very small and cautious increases in your activity, both physical and mental, once you have achieved stability and consistency;
- look at 'what gets in the way of being sensible';
- do whatever is possible to improve your mood. If you suffer from anxiety, panic, or depression, use self-help techniques and/or accept professional help;
- improve your skills in problem solving and communication;
- work on improving relationships;
- get the best you can from today while planning for the future;
- think about the ways in which you will manage the changes that better health may bring. Use problem-solving techniques.

You do not need to put your life on hold, waiting for some 'magic bullet' that will give you a cure. Maybe such a cure will be found, but it is not going to happen in the near future. You can do a great deal meanwhile by using self-help techniques. You deserve to give yourself the best life today, rather than waiting for some possible tomorrow.

Section 3

Special issues

31

Thinking about therapies and therapists, both medical and complementary/ alternative

As we said in Chapter 8, there is no 'magic bullet' that will *cure* CFS/ME. However, most people would still like to believe that there must be something out there that will at least help and so look for a treatment of some kind. Making a choice between the enormous variety of therapies available can be extremely difficult. We thought we could be of most assistance to you if we looked at this subject under three headings:

1. Therapies and therapists in general
2. Medical therapies
3. Alternative and complementary therapies.

Therapies and therapists in general

We are not going to look here at any specific medical, complementary, or alternative treatments. Instead, we are going to talk about the points we believe you should consider and the questions you should ask before embarking on any of them. In this way we hope that you will be able to make informed and sound decisions.

In a condition like CFS/ME in which there are no ready cures but many treatments, it can be difficult to decide what to do for the best:

- Should people with CFS/ME use a drug treatment?

- Should they seek rehabilitative treatment like CBT?

- Should they buy one of the large range of complementary or alternative therapies that are offered?

- Should they just stick with the kind of self-help that we talked about in the previous section or use other treatments as well?

- Is it sensible to 'pick and mix' from all of these?

You will find our answers to these questions at the end of this chapter.

Although your choice will obviously be limited by what is available in your area, by the referrals your own doctor (and perhaps your medical insurance) is willing to support, and by your financial situation, we aim to give you some guidance on how to choose a treatment. We will suggest which aspects of the treatment you should consider and what questions you should ask both yourself and whoever is giving the treatment. Most of what we say can be applied to any treatment, although we accept that there are differences between medical and alternative/complementary treatments.

Why do you want a treatment?

This may seem like a silly question to ask, but people do have very different reasons for seeking treatment. If you are clear about what you want from the treatment it will help you to choose:

- Are you looking for a 'cure'? Do you believe that if you go on looking long enough you will find one? The plain truth is that, so far, *nothing* has yet been found that will reliably *cure* CFS/ME. If that is your hope, we are afraid that you are probably heading for disappointment.

- Are you looking for something that will make you feel better generally, such as a reduction in symptoms?

- Are you looking for help with one or more specific symptoms?

- Are you looking for an increase in energy and an improvement in what you are able to do?

- Are you looking for ongoing support and encouragement?

- Are you unhappy that your family doctor is not offering you any treatment?

Potential benefits of trying any treatment

- You may find it helpful.
- The idea that you are doing something to help yourself may give you a sense of control over the illness.
- Any reduction in symptoms, even if limited, is to be welcomed.

Potential disadvantages of trying any treatment

- If you do improve, you may mistakenly give the credit to the therapy/therapist rather than to what you are doing to help yourself or to the natural progress of the condition. This may reduce your feeling of being able to manage the illness yourself. You may also feel that continued improvement depends on continuing with the treatment.

- If the therapy does not do any good, having your expectations of cure or improvement disappointed may add to your feelings of frustration and hopelessness.

- It may cost you a lot of money (which might be better spent on other things). Indeed, we are concerned that a minority of doctors and therapists do seem to be taking advantage of the desperate or the despairing.

- Treatments that rely on something given to you or something done for you by someone else can be a distraction from the self-help we discuss in this book.

- If there is no improvement, some doctors and therapists may blame the patient—saying that they have not tried hard enough or persisted long enough. While this may sometimes be true, life with CFS/ME is tough enough without being blamed in this way.

- There is a small chance that some treatments could harm you.

Looking at the evidence

In order to make the best choice you will have to consider what evidence there is for the effectiveness of each treatment. In Chapter 1 we talked about the three levels of evidence—the anecdotal reports of other sufferers, the opinion of therapists and doctors based on clinical experience, and the evidence from clinical research:

Anecdotal evidence

Anecdotal reports are the easiest to come by but are also the least reliable. Just because someone you know tells you that such-and-such has helped them (or somebody they know), it does not mean that it will necessarily help you. Do remember that the illnesses of people with CFS/ME vary greatly, so that what helped another person may not do anything for you. Anecdotal evidence can be considered, but on its own it is not the best basis for choice, although it may help you decide whether a particular doctor or therapist has the 'style' you prefer.

Clinical experience

The reported experience of therapists, clinicians, and patients' organizations may be more useful if it is based on the response of many patients to a treatment. However, like anyone else, clinicians, therapists, and those providing accounts of the experience of others can be biased in what they recommend. Bias can be a result of limited experience, strong beliefs, misplaced enthusiasm, and sometimes simple financial gain. Although at first glance this would seem to be good-quality evidence, studies have shown again and again that clinical impression is often not supported by careful research.

Systematic research evidence

The best evidence is that from carefully conducted research which has been designed to avoid such bias as far as possible. The very best evidence comes from clinical trials that have been peer reviewed, published in good journals, and repeated in more than one centre. Unfortunately, there is not very much of this evidence for CFS/ME, although there is some—such as that for CBT.

Asking for evidence

In the first section of this book we talked about the scepticism which is necessary when judging research and the need for a good level of evidence on which to judge drug treatments. This scepticism and judgement of evidence is just as important when thinking about whether a treatment is right for you. You do not need to take anyone's word for it (even if it is a doctor's). You have a right to ask about the quality of the evidence.

Questions you should ask the doctor/therapist (and yourself)

You have a right to question anyone offering treatment before you agree to it. You do not need to be hesitant or embarrassed about doing this:

- What does this treatment offer? Does it match with what you want from it? What evidence is there that this treatment has a good chance of doing this? Has there been any good-quality research on the treatment? Is this an experimental treatment?

- Is this treatment part of a research project? You do not have to be a guinea-pig unless you choose to.

Some people are happy to take part in such things but you may prefer not to.

• Has the doctor/therapist experience of using this treatment in patients with CFS/ME? If so, how many? What results has he/she had with them? Does he/she understand the problems you have?

• What are the risks of side-effects or even of being made worse with this treatment?

• What training and qualifications does the therapist have? (It is not always easy to judge how worthwhile these are for some complementary/alternative therapists.) What does the training involve? How long does it take?

• Does the therapist belong to a professional organization that monitors training and standards of treatment? (Again this is not always easy to judge.) Can that organization enforce standards? Is there a complaints procedure?

• How long is the treatment likely to last? Does the doctor/therapist insist on a minimum number of treatments and if so, why? (Be cautious about this one.)

• If you are paying for the treatment, how much is it going to cost in total (including tests, drugs, etc.)? Think about what you might have to give up in order to afford it. Would you do better spending that money on something that makes your life easier or gives you pleasure? We are aware that some patients spend a great deal of money they can ill afford without being helped.

• What will be the cost in terms of your energy? Would you have to travel to have the treatment?

Would the fatigue of getting there and back as well as having the treatment outweigh any benefits?

- Does the therapist carry proper professional insurance?

- Will the doctor/therapist keep in touch with your usual doctor?

Monitoring results

If after all this you decide to go ahead with a treatment, you do need to monitor if it is helping and how much in order to decide whether to continue. This is why we suggest that you are clear about what you want from it. You may need to try more than just one session or continue with a drug or supplement for a while before you can judge its effectiveness. The doctor/therapist should be able to advise you how long it will be before you could expect to see a result. If after taking this into account you feel worse or it does not seem to be helping, then you have a right to stop. As a rough guide, if you cannot see any significant benefit after six weeks, it would probably be better to stop. Do not let yourself be bullied into continuing if you do not want to. Give yourself a pause. You can then decide whether to continue or to try something else. If you are paying for the treatment, you might decide to use the money in a different way.

Self-help is a treatment

We described self-help techniques earlier in this book. These are intended to help you achieve your own rehabilitation by giving your body the best chance of doing its own healing. They are just as much 'treatments' as any drug or alternative therapy. Do not be trapped into thinking 'If I'm only doing that, then I'm not doing the best for myself.' This applies just as much to the cognitive behaviour and graded exercise therapies which we discuss in the next chapter (which are very similar to self-help, but with expert back-up and support). Research evidence, clinical experience, and anecdotal evidence have shown that, at the present time, these are the most effective treatments available. They are not a cure, but they can improve both your bodily state and your well-being. If you choose to concentrate on them, you will certainly be giving yourself a good chance of improvement. If you choose to add some other form of treatment, chosen sensibly, you may find it helpful. It does not have to be an 'either/or' choice.

Medical therapists and therapies

The general practitioner

Your starting point is likely to be your own doctor. Happily, most people know and trust their general practitioner. Most family doctors offer only ethical and reputable treatment. If you feel that your doctor does not understand your condition or is not giving you the best advice and treatment, do talk about your concerns. If you really cannot sort things out, you may be able to see another doctor in the same practice who has more knowledge or interest in CFS/ME. As a last resort, you may decide to change your family doctor, but do remember that there are disadvantages as well as advantages to starting with someone new.

Specialist doctors

Your own doctor may refer you to a hospital specialist or CFS/ME clinic. Hospital doctors are subject to the scrutiny of their colleagues and are answerable to professional regulatory bodies. These factors make it less likely that they will use treatments that are un-ethical or not based on evidence. Furthermore, in the UK such treatment may well be available free of charge.

There can be advantages in having a specialist diagnosis. It may be comforting to know that you have been checked out by someone really knowledge-able; it may make it easier to obtain benefits. It may be reassuring to feel that you could return if your symptoms change, although not all hospital specialists offer follow-ups after diagnosis.

However, not all doctors treating CFS/ME are using evidence-based treatments. Do be particularly cautious about doctors who are not recommended by your own family doctor, who work on their own, or who are making money from selling treatments. Do make sure that you have satisfied yourself about the questions we suggest you ask before you agree to accept treatment. Do not spend more money than you can afford.

'Doctor shopping'

Some people with CFS/ME feel that if they go on looking long enough and 'shopping around' they will find the 'ideal doctor', someone who will understand both them and their condition and make a significant difference to their illness. On the whole, this is a mistake. Such a search can take up a great deal of time, energy, and money. It may involve them in travelling long distances to see doctors whom they have heard about or had recommended. All of this can actually make their condition worse and will certainly be a distraction from using self-help.

Once you have found a family doctor you are comfortable with, and perhaps had an authoritative diagnosis from a medical specialist, you will probably do better to stick with that and concentrate on working to manage your condition.

Conventional drug therapies

Probably the most important of these are the 'so-called' antidepressant drugs. These are fully described in Chapter 21. For some people they can help to reverse the brain changes that underlie the illness.

The other conventional therapies are largely symptom-relieving drugs such as sedatives to aid sleep and analgesics, which we discussed in Chapters 14 and 16. Used in a sensible way they can be useful. But you might want to try self-help techniques first.

Experimental drug treatments

Some doctors, whether working in a hospital setting or on their own, are experimental in their approach. This may suit you and you might just be lucky enough to find something that really helps. On the other hand, you might find that many of these therapies do not help and may actually have some unpleasant or harmful effects.

If you are being given a treatment of unproven value, it should ideally be as part of a properly evaluated research project. Participating in research can be a way to get better than standard treatment. But remember that you should understand fully what is involved and be asked for your 'informed consent'.

Non-drug treatments

A medical treatment does not have to involve taking a drug. There are also powerful 'non-drug' treatments or therapies. These include such things as cognitive behaviour therapy and graded exercise therapy (see Chapter 32). There are also a variety of medical therapists who can help with specific problems. For example, you could get help from physiotherapists for dealing with deconditioning or specific muscle problems, or you could get psychological therapy from psychiatrists, psychologists, and counsellors for addressing emotional problems.

Complementary/alternative therapists and therapies

These are treatments that lie outside conventional medicine. The distinction between complementary and alternative can be somewhat blurred. Complementary therapies tend to be those that it is suggested are used alongside conventional medicine. Indeed, some doctors have trained in some of these treatments, such as homeopathy and acupuncture. Alternative therapies (as the name suggests), on the other hand, are more likely to be suggested as an alternative to conventional treatment. As we said in Chapter 8, these therapies can range from things that your doctor might be happy to recommend to some that are frankly bizarre and possibly dangerous.

Potential advantages of complementary/alternative treatments

- Complementary/alternative therapies may appeal to you as more 'natural' than mainstream medicine.

- A complementary/alternative therapist may give you more time than a busy doctor is able to offer. Just having someone listening to your problems in a sympathetic way and taking an interest in you as a person (not just as a case) can be helpful. Ongoing support can make managing any illness much easier.

- You may prefer to be able to choose a treatment for yourself rather than having your doctor decide for you.

Potential disadvantages of complementary/alternative treatments

- In general, complementary/alternative therapists are subject to less regulation than doctors. There is, therefore, more opportunity for dubious treatment and unethical practice.

- Alternative therapies usually cost money. Be sure you can afford it.

- There is very little systematic research evidence for the effectiveness of most complementary/alternative therapies. This can make it very hard to judge how likely they are to help you.

- Some complementary/alternative practitioners suggest ideas about CFS/ME that have no scientific basis. They can be confusing and even fanciful. If they suggest that your illness has a simple cause (such as diet or dental fillings), this may be initially encouraging. Unfortunately, it is very unlikely to be the answer. It may also make you feel less confident about what you can do by self-help.

• You may find that your doctor is very dismissive about your use of such therapies.

A few warnings

Whilst there is no doubt that some therapies can help with specific symptoms—for instance, osteopathy or chiropractic can be useful treatments for some back problems—others can have very little value or be potentially dangerous. We are concerned about the number of people with CFS/ME who are advised to use very restricted diets or massive supplements of vitamins or minerals. Some therapists diagnose food sensitivities or allergies by very unscientific methods.

It is worth being very cautious about any therapist who is not willing to make contact with your usual doctor. Be wary of suggestions that you must stop using conventional medicine. In particular, do not stop any conventional medical treatment abruptly (for instance, antidepressant drugs) without first discussing this with your doctor. Do be aware that some herbal remedies can conflict with medically prescribed drugs.

Many of the patients we have talked with report that they have expended a great deal of time, energy, and money on alternative therapies (probably more than they could afford of all three) without getting any real benefit.

Deciding to try a complementary/alternative treatment

As with so many other people with CFS/ME, you may find some of these therapists and therapies helpful. In spite of the cautions we have highlighted, we are certainly not saying that you should not use them. Indeed there is *some* evidence that *some* therapies (such as homeopathy) can help *some* patients with *some* of their symptoms. Something like massage that you enjoy may make you feel a little better, at least for a while. All that we suggest is that you should think carefully about which ones you choose and consider the evidence for their effectiveness. Just because therapists tell you that something is effective does not mean that you have to take their advice or believe that it is true without them having given you good evidence. We have included a book in the reading list (Appendix 4) which could give you some guidance on choosing a therapy and a therapist.

You may already have found that there is a good deal of pressure put on you by relatives, friends, or other people with CFS/ME to try complementary/alternative therapies. Some of these people can suggest that if you are not trying these therapies then you are not trying to get better. You may also find that other people read something in the paper about the latest 'cure' and insist that you try it. You are the one with the illness and you have a right to choose what you do—you do not need to give in to these pressures.

Summary—where has all this got us?

Of course you would like to feel that there is some treatment out there that will make you feel better or improve your situation. Trying some of them may help you or make you feel more in control of your illness. Finding someone, whether a doctor or a complementary/alternative therapist, who will look at you as a complete person (rather than just a collection of symptoms) and give you ongoing support can be very comforting.

At the beginning of this chapter we asked if people with CFS/ME should try drug treatments, rehabilitative treatments, complementary/alternative therapies, or just stick to self-help and if it would be sensible to 'pick and mix' from a variety of treatments. Our answer to those questions is that you should first think about what you can do for yourself. If, after careful consideration, you want to try a treatment as well, then do so. You can continue self-help techniques as well. However, if you are trying a mix of treatments, it can be hard to decide which one helps.

All that we hope is that you will take some of our warnings to heart and be cautious and selective about which treatments you choose. Becoming preoccupied with a search for the 'perfect' treatment that will solve all your problems is likely to be expensive, exhausting, and fruitless. It may also distract you from what you can do to help yourself.

Trying out treatments, whether medical or complementary/alternative techniques, can have advantages and disadvantages. Think first about what you are looking for from a treatment. You are likely to make a better choice if you look carefully at the evidence for the effectiveness of any treatment. You have a right to question the doctor or therapist before you agree to take part. You need to monitor the effect of any treatment in order to decide if it is worth continuing. Do not spend more money than you can really afford. Having a treatment does not mean that you should stop using self-help techniques—you can certainly use both.

32

Cognitive behaviour therapy and graded exercise therapy

In previous chapters we have talked about cognitive behaviour therapy (CBT) and its use in various ways. (Cognitive, by the way, is a word describing thoughts and beliefs.) In this chapter we explain in more detail what it is (and what it is not!) and how it can be used to help people with CFS/ME and also those suffering from anxiety, panic, phobias, or depression.

The ideas behind CBT

CBT is based on the observation that the way you think about an illness and the way you cope with it influences its outcome. Your initial reactions to this idea might be:

1. Doesn't everyone think the same way about his or her illness?

2. How can thinking and coping behaviour affect a physical illness?

3. How could you change your thinking anyway?

Doesn't everyone think the same way about his or her illness?

People do not all think in the same way—look at the different ways they vote in an election! The more ambiguous the situation, the greater the variation in what people think about it.

Consider this example. You are in bed alone and you hear a noise downstairs. You do not know exactly what it is. What do you think? You might think it is an intruder—or you might decide it is just the cat. These are very different thoughts with very different effects on how you feel and how you behave. We probably do not need to emphasize to you that CFS/ME is an illness surrounded by misunderstanding and uncertainty—a condition likely to produce a variety of interpretations.

How can thinking and coping behaviour affect a physical illness?

Thinking affects your mood, your behaviour, and your physiological (bodily) state. To continue our example, if you think that the noise is an intruder you are likely to be anxious (mood), jump out of bed (behaviour), and develop a faster heart rate (bodily state). These reactions will be the same whether the noise was an actual intruder or just the cat! It is your thoughts and beliefs that determine your reaction—not the reality. Persistently inaccurate thinking can lead to poor coping and to adverse emotional, behavioural, and physiological states. For instance, if a person worries constantly that things will go wrong they will be chronically anxious, tend to avoid doing things, and be in a physiological state of tension and arousal.

These effects not only alter how you feel but can influence the course of illness. There is now increasing evidence that how patients think about diseases such as heart attacks and cancer influence how long they live. The way this works may be partly by influencing what treatment they seek and how they cope (for example, by getting fitter or by taking to bed). There may also be direct effects on the body—for example, the functioning of the nervous and immune systems can be influenced by mood state and coping behaviour.

How could you change your thinking anyway?

A central tenet of CBT is that you can choose what to think. You can look for evidence (for example, by going downstairs and having a look and deciding that it was not an intruder but the cat knocking something over). The therapist helps, not by a process of brainwashing, but by support and guidance. You are the one who decides what to think.

What is CBT?

CBT was originally developed over thirty years ago by an American psychiatrist, Aaron Beck, as a treatment for depression. Since then, CBT has been adapted to treat many other conditions, both psychological and physical. There is a substantial body of research evidence that demonstrates its effectiveness.

CBT for depression

People suffering from depression are typically low in mood. They also tend to have negative and inaccurate thoughts and beliefs. Specifically, they are likely to regard themselves, their future, and their circumstances in a very negative manner. For example, they may think that they are a worthless person, in a hopeless predicament, and with no future. This inaccurate and distorted thinking was long thought to be simply a *result* of their depression. Beck's innovation was to suggest and demonstrate that this thinking could also be a *cause* of their depression and that by changing their thinking patients could get better.

CBT works by helping patients to develop more accurate and helpful ways of thinking about themselves, their situation, and their future. This does not simply mean adopting equally inaccurate positive thinking, but rather getting evidence to test out alternative thoughts and beliefs and seeing which of these reflect the real world in the most accurate way (in our example by going downstairs to see what is happening).

What happens during CBT treatment for depression?

During the treatment sessions, the therapist helps the patients to clarify how they are thinking and coping now and to consider different ways of thinking and behaving. Between treatment sessions patients carry out 'homework' tasks. For instance, they may be set the task of catching and recording their thoughts about themselves ('I am a failure'). Once these thoughts have been identified, the patient can be helped to challenge them by looking at alternative views (for example, 'some things I have tried to do have failed, but others have succeeded. This does not make me a failure as a person.'). Finally, the evidence for each is examined (by reviewing past achievements, asking other people, or trying out new endeavours).

CBT for anxiety and panic

Once the value of CBT in depression was established, psychiatrists and psychologists went on to identify inaccurate and distorted thinking in patients with other problems such as anxiety, panic, and phobias. For example, people who panic tend to 'catastrophize' physical symptoms (a twinge of chest pain is interpreted as 'I'm having a heart attack') and consequently pay excessive attention to minor bodily symptoms. A person with phobia tends to exaggerate risk (for example, someone who fears flying may think 'there is a 90 per cent chance that a plane will crash' and consequently avoid flying).

Versions of CBT were developed to help patients overcome such problems. Again, these are based on identifying the thoughts and the ways of thinking associated with such states and then finding more realistic alternatives. Patients are encouraged to challenge negative thoughts and catastrophic interpretations of symptoms.

CBT for physical illnesses

In recent years, forms of CBT have been devised for people suffering from a wide range of physical conditions such as chronic pain, cancer, and the after-effects of a heart attack. Using CBT, patients can be helped to cope more effectively, to improve their ability to function and their quality of life. For instance, someone with chronic pain might be helped to return to previously enjoyed activities in spite of their pain.

CBT for CFS/ME

What it is not

Before we go on to talk about what it *is*, it may help if we spell out what it is *not*:

- It is not another way of saying that CFS/ME is 'all in the mind'.
- It does not imply that a person with CFS/ME is failing to try.
- It does not imply that the only reason a person with CFS/ME stays ill is because of inaccurate beliefs about their illness.
- It is not 'a programme of ruthlessly increased exercise imposed on helpless CFS/ME victims'.

What it is

CBT for CFS/ME is not new. It was first used more than ten years ago and since then there has been a good deal of research to refine the techniques. Therapists have listened to their patients and tried to learn from them. CBT is now being offered in many centres and the therapists can be psychiatrists, psychologists, or trained nurse counsellors. We cannot emphasize enough that CBT should be a collaboration between the patients and the therapist—it is not something *imposed* on them. Patients are treated as individuals. Therapists use a very holistic approach, looking at all the factors involved for each individual. The aim is to achieve the maximum degree of rehabilitation and to improve patients' functioning as well as aiming for a better quality of life for the individual.

In Section 2 we outlined all the things that people with CFS/ME can do to help themselves. We know from experience that many people find it hard to do this on their own. It is much easier to undertake and stick to such a programme with expert guidance and back-up. It can be a great help to have a therapist who understands about CFS/ME giving you guidance and support. There are bound to be times when you come up against problems and have doubts about what you are doing. Talking things through with the therapist can make quite a difference. It can also be very thera-peutic to have someone to whom you can report your successes, particularly if that person can understand the difficulties you may have had to surmount to achieve such success.

What happens during a course of CBT treatment

The typical CBT course normally involves about 16 sessions lasting one hour each. They are usually scheduled weekly to begin with, but perhaps every fortnight later on. There may also be a follow-up session some months later to check on progress. Patients are often expected to do 'homework' between sessions. A typical course of treatment might be structured like this:

Stages of therapy	Sessions
1. Assessment, formulation, and goal setting	1–3
2. Stabilization of activity/rest/sleep Re-evaluation of illness beliefs Experiment of a gradual increase in activity	4–10
3. Reviewing unhelpful attitudes	8–12
4. Problem solving practical difficulties	10–14
5. Review and planning for the future	12–16

Assessment

It is usual for a medical assessment to have already been done. The CBT therapist needs to build up a complete picture of the patient, looking at *all* aspects—not just the biomedical. Such an assessment might include looking at:

- Current problems—symptoms, life difficulties, severity of fatigue, and current level of disability.

- Cognitions—patients' beliefs about the illness, their understanding of the cause of the symptoms, the significance of an increase in symptoms after exercise, their 'worst fears', how they believe the illness should be managed, and their hopes and fears concerning rehabilitative treatment. Patients may be asked to record their thoughts in a diary format.

- Mood—the impact of the illness on their emotions, frustration, possible anxiety, or depression, and so on.

- Behaviour—how patients cope with fatigue, how they attempt to relieve symptoms. A detailed account of the patient's current life will be examined by going through a typical day hour by hour, or by asking the patient to keep a diary for a week or two. This record is useful both in providing a baseline and in identifying patterns of activity, rest, and sleep.

- Interpersonal and social factors—looking at interpersonal, occupational, or financial factors that might be potential blocks to recovery. It is often very helpful to discover the views and beliefs of partners or family—what they think about the illness and the best way of managing it. The therapist may seek to talk with such 'significant others'.

Stabilizing activity/rest/sleep

Using the data gathered during the assessment, the therapist would now seek to help the patient find out if he/she can start to get the illness under control. The first step is to try to adopt a consistent pattern of activity, rest, and sleep that can be kept up without exacerbating symptoms. This may often involve an individual doing rather less to begin with and resting in a more structured way.

Re-evaluation of illness beliefs

During the assessment process, the therapist will have learnt what the patient believes about his/her illness and how best to manage it. Rather than saying 'This belief is inaccurate' the therapist would encourage patients to try some behavioural experiments to check the accuracy of such beliefs for themselves and then to look at other possible beliefs. Such initial beliefs might include 'Rest is the only way of managing CFS/ME' or 'Any increase in symptoms means that I am harming myself.'

Experiment of a gradual increase in activity

Once a consistent level of activity, both physical and mental, has been achieved, the therapist and patient together can work out some specific goals of increased activity and decide on the small steps towards achieving them.

Reviewing unhelpful attitudes

Throughout the treatment, the therapist will aim to help patients see that improvement can be achieved by their own efforts and to help them gain increasing confidence in their ability to function. A good therapist will help them take responsibility for their recovery without ever implying that they are to blame for their current predicament.

After patients have started to increase their level of activity, many of them become increasingly concerned about the significance of increasing fatigue and/or muscle pain. The therapist will review with the patient the evidence for and against the belief that they have a sinister significance. This is also a time to look at general attitudes such as perfectionism with an 'all-or-nothing' approach to activity, or the view that 'I should always do what other people ask of me'. Such attitudes often lead to large swings in activity and make it difficult to try the behavioural experiment of a careful and graded increase in activity.

Problem solving practical difficulties

Being ill produces problems, but getting better can do so too. The therapist is likely to help the patient to master the techniques of problem solving and then to apply them to current problems, as well as looking at problems that may crop up as the patient's condition improves. This may be a time to look at the specific difficulties that could occur if a return to work seems possible.

Review and planning for the future

By the end of therapy, the therapist and the patient should have together worked out and agreed a 'formulation' of what the illness is and what works for the patient in managing it. The patient is often asked to produce a written document which includes this formulation and a list of what he or she has learnt from the therapy. Therapist and patient together may produce practical guidelines on how rehabilitation can continue after the CBT treatment has ended and how to cope with a possible relapse.

Summary

CBT for CFS/ME is about rehabilitation, not cure. It seeks to help individuals find the best ways of managing themselves to produce an increased quality of life and have a good chance of decreasing disability. It also helps patients to identify and deal with 'what gets in the way of being sensible'. CBT is a 'tool', not a rigid form of treatment. It can be adapted to an individual's needs and concentrate on the areas that will produce the most benefit for that individual— whether a physical improvement or an increase in their quality of life. You may recognize that it is very much the same as what was discussed in Section 2.

Does CBT work for people with CFS/ME?

Yes, it does seem to help. It is not a cure, but research trials, clinical experience, and anecdotal evidence have shown that about two-thirds of patients who take part in such a programme achieve an increased ability to do things. It has also been shown that it can decrease symptoms and lead to an improved quality of life.

Graded exercise therapy (GET)

GET is similar in many ways to CBT, but it concentrates more on stabilizing and then increasing *physical* activity, rather than on general activity as in CBT. The rate of increase is not imposed on the patient—the patient will not be encouraged to move on to the next stage in the programme until the previous stage has been assimilated and symptoms have returned to an acceptable level. In the early stages the increase in activity will be a very small one. Patients are likely to be asked to start with 5 to 15 minutes of gentle exercise. This amount can then be increased by one or two minutes at a time (depending on progress) up to a maximum of 30 minutes a day. Like CBT, it should be a collaboration between patient and therapist—increases are not imposed on a patient and there is no insistence on an increase every week.

As in CBT, the patients' thoughts and beliefs do need to be taken into consideration. Difficulties and fears about increasing physical activity can be openly discussed.

There is evidence from clinical trials that GET can be helpful for some patients. It may well be that those it helps most are those suffering most from the effects of deconditioning. It may also be possible that at least some of the benefit comes from giving patients back a sense of self-efficacy.

'So-called' CBT and GET

Unfortunately, there are some therapies that are being offered under the name of CBT and GET which are *not* collaborations between patients and therapists. Some health professionals have read briefly about CBT and GET and offer a version under those names. As with any other therapy, you have a right to question the therapist before starting the therapy. We hope that you now have a much better idea of what the real versions imply.

Cognitive behaviour therapy (CBT) is a very effective tool to help people suffering from depression, anxiety, and panic. It can also help people suffering from many physical illnesses including CFS/ME. It is not a 'cure' but it can lead to an improvement in functioning. It is not something imposed on patients and should be a collaboration between a therapist and a patient. It should be tailored to an individual.

Graded exercise therapy (GET) is somewhat similar, but concentrates more on an increase in exercise rather than on activities in general.

33
Children with CFS/ME

It is not only adults who can get CFS/ME. It is a sad fact that children and young people can suffer from it as well. Their symptoms can be very similar to those experienced by adults, though they may not talk about being fatigued in quite the same way. Like adults, the onset of illness may be acute following a viral-type illness (such as glandular fever) or may be more gradual. As we have said before, the label CFS/ME probably covers more than one condition, so your child's illness may be very different from that of another child with the same diagnosis.

Obviously, an illness like this is intensely worrying and distressing for parents. Not knowing what to do for the best can add enormously to the load that parents have to bear. We hope that if you are a parent of a child with CFS/ME you will have read the earlier sections of this book and so feel a little more knowledgeable about what will help.

Diagnosis

The way CFS/ME is diagnosed in children is much the same as that described for adults in Chapter 4. The major difference is that it is now agreed that it is appropriate to make a diagnosis in a child after three months of illness, rather than wait until after a damaging six months of illness.

The same sort of questions, examinations, and diagnostic tests are used to exclude other conditions that could produce similar symptoms. Some family doctors may call in other health professionals—a paediatrician or a child psychiatrist or psychologist—to assist them in making the diagnosis and exclude other conditions.

As with adults, these other conditions can include emotional problems. In children these include anxiety about going to school (school phobia), anorexia nervosa, and depression. (Yes, children can suffer from depression.) As a parent you may feel that your child's illness could not be emotional. However, it is worth being open to the possibility that he or she has one of these conditions, which can produce similar physical symptoms. The advantage of making these diagnoses is that they lead to specific treatments.

Do not be too alarmed if your child is given a diagnosis of CFS/ME. In our experience the cases that have been given attention in the newspapers and on television are unusually severe. You really do have grounds for reasonable optimism.

Prognosis

Studies that have examined the outcome of children who have received a diagnosis of CFS/ME show that, in general, the outlook is good for children and certainly better than for adults. This seems to be especially true if the children and their families have received good advice and help early in the illness. Although recovery may take some time, the majority of children are much improved by two years after onset. Even if your child has been ill for a longer time than this, effective rehabilitation is possible. Most children do recover and go on to lead normal lives.

Getting help

The help that parents and children get from their general practitioners and other health professionals can be crucial in achieving a good outcome for a child with CFS/ME. That is why it is so important to establish a positive working relationship with them. You might want to refer to Chapter 25 on how to get the best from your doctor.

You may feel that your family doctor does not fully understand your child's problems. If you have concerns about this, express them calmly and clearly. If you are still unhappy, see if there is another doctor in the practice who has greater interest and expertise in childhood CFS/ME and your child's individual difficulties. If all else fails, you might want to change doctors, but do be aware that this means starting again with somebody new.

You may also feel that if only you could find the right specialist your child could be made better. In reality, most paediatricians are familiar with CFS/ME and there is probably little to be gained from seeking second and further opinions. If you do decide to seek further opinions, beware of the negative effect that multiple opinions and fragmented management can have on your child's care.

It is not only the doctor who can help, but also the other people who may become involved in the care of a child who is ill—the multidisciplinary team of teachers, educational psychologists, education authorities, social services, and so on. Do use your experience as a parent to keep them informed of your child's difficulties, needs, and progress. Teachers or doctors may only see the child for a short time and not be aware of some of the difficulties. For instance, teachers may not be aware that your child has problems with memory and concentration, or that mental activity can be as tiring as physical.

Self-help—achieving a balance

So what can parents do to give their child the best chance of recovery? Everything we have said about good management in Section 2 applies just as much to children and young people as it does to adults.

The mainstays of management are to ensure that the diagnosis is correct, to address problems such as depression, to establish a manageable routine, and then to work gradually towards a return to normal activity.

However, because children are much more dependent on the adults around them, are growing and developing and are still in education, they have special needs. In order to help them most effectively, parents have to help their children to achieve a balance in a number of areas.

It is also important for the parents themselves to work towards a balance between pushing children and treating them as 'poor darlings' who must have everything done for them.

Balancing the day

Children with CFS/ME often lose the usual daily routine and may need guidance and help to structure their day. The overall aim is to establish a manageable and regular routine of sleeping, eating, and activity.

Sleeping

It is important to maintain or re-establish a regular pattern of sleep. If children have slept badly, it can be very tempting to let them sleep on later and later into the morning. It is much better to stick to a regular, normal waking time. If this is not done, children with CFS/ME can end up sleeping most of the day and being awake most of the night, which is something to try to avoid. Our advice on improving sleep in Chapter 14 applies to children as well as adults. As with adults, a small dose of a sedative antidepressant can help with sleep problems, though this is something you would need to discuss with your child's doctor.

Eating and diet

Regular meal times are also important. Anything that keeps a normal rhythm going during the day will be helpful. Try to stick to normal meal times (although it may suit some children better to include small healthy snacks at set times between meals). Allowing 'grazing' just when a child feels like it is probably not a good idea.

Growing children need good food. Their meals should include all the food groups (as discussed in Chapter 16). Whatever you may read or hear, most children do not need special diets. However, calcium is essential for the development of strong bones, so if it has really been *proved* that a child is intolerant of milk products, supplements of calcium may be needed. Discuss this with your doctor.

Balancing activity with rest and relaxation

Children need both rest and activity for health. This balance is likely to be upset by the illness. The best approach is to begin by establishing a pattern of rest and activity that your child can manage on a daily basis. Time-limited periods of activity (both physical and mental) alternated with good-quality rest, spread evenly through the day, are probably best. The length of the periods of activity initially will obviously depend on just how much an individual child can manage. The aim is to achieve a programme which does not increase symptoms too much and which can be managed every day in a consistent way. Do read Chapter 12 on 'Balancing rest and activity'.

Prolonged bedrest, in particular, is to be avoided. It has an effect on the body called deconditioning, which causes weak muscles and other problems (as we discussed in Chapter 14). Complete bedrest quickly produces deconditioning, which is to be avoided. Whilst some time in bed may be necessary for a number of days after an acute illness, this rest period should be kept brief. It has been plausibly argued that some of the symptoms that children with CFS/ME experience may in fact be the result of too much time in bed, resulting in deconditioning. Passive exercise with the parent helping the child to move their limbs in bed can be a start towards normal movements.

Initially, a child may need to be encouraged to get out of bed and walk, even if it is only for a few steps at intervals during the day. Later on, longer distances and more vigorous exercise should be possible. Exercise periods should be planned so that they are within the child's current capacity and end before the child becomes too tired. As with adults, pacing is vital— stopping before fatigue becomes excessive.

Good-quality rest is also important. The best rest comes when the child is really relaxed, in body and in mind (see Chapter 13). Even quite young children can be taught how to relax (one of the authors taught her own young children). Complete relaxation can also ease symptoms. Thrashing around in bed is likely to make problems of pain and malaise worse. If you can teach children how to relax you will be giving them a tool that will be useful to them for the rest of their lives.

Rehabilitation

Once such a stable routine is established, rehabilitation can begin. The lengths of the periods of activity (both physical and mental) can then be increased very gradually. The pace of increase should be within the child's capacity and manageable. A physiotherapist may be able to help here.

Balancing appropriate discipline and too much control

Even quite small children need to feel that they have some control over themselves and their lives. It is not always easy to find the right balance between discipline and allowing a child to have choices, especially when that child is ill. This may be especially hard for parents who experienced similar difficulties when they were children. This ability to identify with your child can be both an advantage and a disadvantage. It is an advantage in helping you understand your child and how they might be feeling. It can, however, be a disadvantage when it comes to imposing discipline, for example about attending school.

Striking a balance can be difficult. Nevertheless, it is important to your child's recovery and general development and something worth working at. It is an area where the observations of a more 'objective' professional may be helpful.

Social contact

This is a vital need for a child's normal development. Loneliness and isolation can certainly add to any child's distress, so it is important to explore ways in which social contact can be kept up. For example, a child with CFS/ME will almost certainly be able to cope with *short* visits from friends. You can help by making it easy and pleasant for visitors (a reputation for providing wonderful cakes helps!). If your child cannot cope with even short visits, then you could explore other methods—telephone calls (though you may need to ration the time spent on the phone), letters, or postcards to friends. These days many children can use computers so e-mail could be another way of making contact, but there again you might need to limit time spent on the computer. A small kitchen timer can be useful to limit the time spent on an activity.

Education

Obviously, an illness like this can have a major effect on a child's education. There are no hard and fast rules on how to deal with this—each child must be assessed as an individual. It is a good idea to talk to teachers right from the beginning to plan the best for the child and to get as much cooperation as possible, aiming for a flexible approach. A return to school is the aim, even if only part-time at first.

When the time comes to return to school, this is best planned in advance. Doing too much, too soon can lead to a setback and to loss of confidence. It may be better, therefore, to start with a part-time return— a few lessons a week in school can help to maintain a normal life and to keep up social contact. Academic education and examinations can wait for a while. It is surprising how quickly children can catch up once they recover.

Even though a child is eager to return to school, absence may lead to anxiety about coping when he or she goes back. It can be helpful to bring this out into the open and discuss it. If your child does talk about problems about returning to school, you can help him or her to overcome these using a technique called 'problem solving', which is described in Chapter 24. (We have found that children as young as five can understand and use problem solving.)

In some cases when school attendance does not seem possible, home tuition may be considered for a time. This has advantages in helping the child who is too ill to keep up with school, but has the major disadvantage of not providing the normal school social environment. It is best used, therefore, only for a limited period. The school health team (nurse and doctor) can be of great help in planning your child's return to school.

Emotions and emotional problems

Adults with CFS/ME can have emotional problems as part of the illness. Children are no different. Children may feel frightened, resentful, grieving, anxious, and angry. They may already be facing the challenges of adolescence and demands of school, which are further complicated by the illness. They may find it hard to express these feelings. Furthermore, the expression of their distress may get all mixed up with feeling physically unwell.

It will help them if they can talk about their pre-dicament and what they are feeling about it. They may find it easier to talk freely to someone outside the immediate family, so contact with a nurse, counsellor, or child psychologist can be useful.

Openness within the family is also important. Some parents feel that they should try to maintain a calm and optimistic manner at all times so as 'not to upset' the child. However, this can lead to children with CFS/ME believing that their feelings (which may be neither calm nor optimistic) are not important or that it is bad to express them. This only adds to their problems.

If depression or anxiety is a block to progress, this is best treated. As with adults, both psychological help and medication for depression may have an important role in helping them to recover.

Self-esteem

Any illness can undermine a child's sense of self-esteem. You can help here—setting small achievable targets and giving praise for even small successes will be important.

Teenagers, in particular, care about their appearance. You may be able to help them with that. (Could you arrange for a visiting hairdresser or get a supply of suitable mail order catalogues from which to choose new clothes?)

Families

It is difficult and distressing for the whole family when a child has a prolonged illness, especially a poorly understood one. Inevitably, there is likely to be an effect on the whole family. Parents suffer distress, worry, and fear for the future and sometimes guilt if the child does not improve. The strain of dealing with a child with CFS/ME can also put stress on the parents' own relationship, particularly if they hold differing views on how the child should be managed. Relatives can sometimes interfere and cause problems. It will be best for the child if you can talk about the problems, both between yourselves and perhaps also with professionals who can help.

Other children in the family may also feel the effects of their sibling's illness. They may feel anxious about their brother or sister, while at the same time feeling resentment at the increased attention that the parents are giving to that child—perhaps feeling that they themselves are being neglected. This can disturb the balance of relationships to the extent that the whole family needs help—not just the child that is ill.

Looking after yourself

Being a parent of a child with CFS/ME is a great strain. You cannot keep it up all day, every day, without it taking its toll on you. This is especially true if your child's difficulties awaken in you unhappy memories from your own childhood, if you feel they are reflecting badly on your ability as a parent, or if you feel the professionals are not helping. You need to look after yourself as well as your child. Do not feel guilty if, at times, you feel resentful at the way your child's illness has changed your life. Try to build in breaks for yourself, even if it is only just for an hour or two each day. That will ease the burden on you a little and help you to stand back from your problems for a while. You might even want to get some support from a councillor for yourself. Your health and emotional well-being are vital to your child; look after them.

Good management from the earliest possible moment will give a child with CFS/ME the best chance of improvement and ultimate recovery. This is likely to involve:

- achieving a balance in their daily life and planning rehabilitation;

- re-establishing regular sleep;

- regular eating and a balanced diet;

- planning periods of physical and mental activity balanced with good-quality rest;

- encouraging appropriate levels of exercise that are increased very gradually;

- keeping schooling and social contact going and working towards a full return;

- dealing positively with emotional problems.

Remember, the welfare of the whole family needs to be looked after in addition to that of the child who is ill. Look after yourself if you are a parent and use all the help you can get.

Appendices

Appendix 1
Medical glossary

If you or a family member suffer from CFS/ME, it is likely that you may come across some medical terms you do not understand, perhaps things you hear from your doctor or that you read in medical reports, textbooks, or research papers. We are well aware that doctors are inclined to use 'doctor speak' and forget that their audience may not understand some of their language. Sometimes a word used medically has a rather different meaning than when it is used in ordinary speech. The following is a brief list of some of the more commonly used terms, with definitions taken mostly from the Oxford Concise Medical Dictionary.

acute Describing a disease of rapid onset, severe symptoms, and brief duration (compare this with chronic)

adrenal glands Two endocrine glands situated on top of the kidneys. They produce hormones including adrenaline and cortisol

adrenaline A hormone which prepares the body for 'fight, flight, or freeze' and has widespread effects on circulation, the muscles, and sugar metabolism

antidepressants Drugs that have proven benefit in people with depressive disorder. They also have wider actions on pain, sleep, appetite, and energy. 'Antidepressant' is a misleading name for these 'brain tonics'

arthralgia Pain in a joint

autonomic nervous system The part of the nervous system responsible for the control of bodily functions that are not consciously directed, such as regular beating of the heart, intestinal movements, sweating, salivation, etc.

biopsy The removal of a small piece of living tissue for microscopic examination

biopsychosocial An approach that takes into account biological, psychological, and social factors

cerebral Of the brain

chronic Describing an illness that has gone on for a long time. It does not imply anything about its severity (compare this with acute)

circadian rhythms Regular cyclic changes within the period of about a day which govern many vital functions such as sleep, feeding, metabolism, and the secretion of many hormones

coeliac disease A condition in which the small intestine fails to digest and absorb food. It is due to a sensitivity of the intestinal lining to a protein contained in gluten (found in wheat, barley, and rye)

cognitive function The mental processes involved in memory, concentration, and attention

cohort A group of people chosen for a research project

cortisol A hormone produced and released by the adrenal glands. It is important for the normal response to any stress or infection

cryptic Something concealed or of unknown origin

cytokines Chemicals produced by cells of the immune system

debility Weakness or feebleness

endocrine system Glands that manufacture hormones and secrete them directly into the bloodstream. They include the pituitary, thyroid, parathyroid, and adrenal glands, as well as the ovaries and testes

endogenous Arising within or derived from the body

enterovirus Any virus that enters the body through the gastrointestinal tract and multiplies there

enzyme A protein that is essential for normal functioning and development of bodily systems

epidemiology The study of the occurrence, pattern, and control of diseases in populations

exogenous The opposite of endogenous—originating outside of the body

fasciculation Muscle twitching, seen as a flicker of movement under the skin

heterogeneous Not all the same, composed of different types

hormone A substance that is produced in one part of the body, passes into the bloodstream, and is carried to other organs or tissues where it regulates their functioning

HPA axis The system connecting and including the hypothalamus, the pituitary gland, and the adrenal glands. It is central to the response to stress

hyper- A prefix meaning over (as in physically above) or higher than normal

hypersomnia Sleeping more than normal

hypertension Blood pressure higher than normal

hypo- A prefix meaning under or less than normal

hypoglycaemia A deficiency of glucose in the blood-stream causing muscular weakness and incoordination, mental confusion, and sweating

hypoperfusion Blood flow less than normal

hypotension Blood pressure less than normal

hypothalamus A region of the brain below the thalamus. It controls the pituitary gland which lies below it and regulates body temperature, thirst, hunger and eating, water balance, and sexual function

iatrogenic Refers to a condition which has resulted from medical treatment, as either an unforeseen or inevitable side-effect

idiopathic Describing a condition the cause of which is unknown

immune system The organs responsible for immunity

immunity The body's ability to resist infection

libido Sexual interest and drive

magnetic resonance imaging (MRI) A method of obtaining high-quality pictures of the inside of the body using high-powered magnets rather than X-rays

medically unexplained Describing a condition or set of symptoms whose cause cannot be identified by standard medical tests. This does not mean that no cause exists, merely that no cause has been identified

melatonin A hormone produced by the pineal gland, which helps to synchronize the body to the 24-hour night/day rhythm (circadian rhythm)

mental Relating to or affecting the mind

multiple sclerosis (MS) A chronic relapsing disease of the nervous system. The myelin sheaths surrounding nerves in the brain and spinal cord are damaged, affecting the function of the nerves involved

myalgia Pain in the muscles

neuroendocrine The system of dual control of certain activities of the body by means of nerves and circulating hormones

neurotransmitter A chemical substance released from nerve endings to transmit impulses to other nerves —the chemical messengers in the brain

osteoporosis Loss of bony tissue, resulting in bones that are brittle and liable to fracture. A diet with adequate calcium and exercise, and hormone replacement therapy for post-menopausal women, can help to prevent it

palpitation An awareness of an irregularity in the heartbeat

paresthesia Numbness or tingling sensations, sometimes called pins and needles

pharmaceutical Relating to drugs used medically

pituitary gland The master endocrine responsible for producing a range of hormones some of which regulate the secretion of hormones from other glands

placebo A medicine or treatment that is ineffective but may help to relieve a condition because the patient has faith in its powers. New drugs are tested against placebos in clinical trials

plasma The straw-coloured fluid in which the blood cells are suspended

psychiatric Relating to psychiatry

psychiatry A branch of medicine that treats patients whose condition is, or was previously thought to be, 'mental'. It is increasingly apparent that these conditions are disturbances of brain function. For example, patients with depression have altered levels of certain neurotransmitters

psychological Relating to psychology

psychology The science and study of the mind, emotion, behaviour, and mental processes

RNA (ribonucleic acid) A chemical found in cells that helps to make proteins

somatic Relating to the body rather than the mind

somatization Refers to a process whereby emotional distress produces physical complaints

somatization disorder A chronic condition characterized by multiple recurrent physical symptoms that are unexplained by identifiable disease and often attributed to somatization

stress Anything that leads to a stress response in the person exposed to it. Stress may be physical (such as noise), psychological (such as worry about work), or social (such as personal attacks). Chronic stress may lead to the development of illnesses such as depression and CFS/ME

T-cells (T-lymphocytes) White blood cells which are part of the immune system

thyroid gland A large endocrine gland situated in the base of the neck. It is concerned with the regulation of the metabolic rate by the secretion of thyroid hormone

virology The study and science of viruses

Appendix 2
Keeping a diary

During the second part of this book, we mentioned some very different kinds of diaries that can be very helpful to you at different stages of your illness. Here are more details about them.

When you start a pacing programme

Keeping an activity diary for two or three weeks can often be a good start to working out a 'pacing programme'. The information from it often shows you how the way that you are managing your day affects how you are feeling. The simplest way is to use a notebook with one page per day. It is a good idea to carry it round with you and enter things as they happen—if you wait till the end of the day to write it up you may well forget quite a lot.

The basic idea is to keep a record of all of your activities (both physical and mental), how long they took, and how you are feeling both physically and emotionally.

You need four columns:

1. *Time*—when you started an activity and when you stopped, so you can know how long you continued
2. *Activity*—both physical and mental activities
3. *How you are feeling physically*—your level of fatigue, malaise, pain, etc.
4. *How you are feeling emotionally*—happy or sad, satisfied or frustrated, etc.

After a while you will probably be able to spot some patterns, such as the 'roller-coaster'. For instance, if you record a day during which you mostly felt very unwell physically and rather low emotionally, you may well notice that that day came after one or more days when you regularly pushed yourself to exhaustion. It is very typical of CFS/ME that the bad effects of getting too tired do not show up until the next day or even the day after that. You may also notice how getting exhausted can leave you feeling in very low spirits.

This sort of diary keeping will help give you some data about how long you can keep up various activities without getting too exhausted—you will have a much better idea of what the right 'bite size' is for you at the moment. You will also get some data to help you spread out your activities throughout the day and throughout the week. It is likely that you will be surprised to find that some activities that you did not think of as particularly strenuous do tire you more than you realized. You may then decide that these need to be rationed for the time being.

We do not suggest that you should go on keeping such a diary for very long; in fact, we think that that can be counterproductive. The process can be tedious and it may make you concentrate too much on symptom scanning and so notice your symptoms much more. However, it can be very helpful at the beginning of your 'pacing programme'. You may find that going back to it for a week or two is useful if you find yourself getting a bit 'off-course' in your pacing.

What gets in the way of being sensible?

In Chapter 20 we talked about catching your thoughts just as you are about to start an activity or when you decide to continue it. This can often give you far greater insight into why you are doing things. Just trying to remember these thoughts is often not very successful. It is often better to carry a small notebook in your pocket and write your thoughts down as they happen. After a while you will probably be able to spot the things that push you into doing too much or too little.

Achievements and happiness diary

It can often be very helpful to keep a diary in which you record only your moments of pleasure, satisfaction, or mastery. Recording what you are 'getting right' can make it easier to identify the moments when you are achieving a good balance between rest and activity as well as the sort of things that improve your quality of life. Building on successes is always a good idea.

Often when people are unwell they tend to concentrate more on what is wrong with their lives than what is right. They tend to forget the good times because the bad times are so much more memorable.

Keeping a diary that focuses on the good times does help to keep things in proportion.

Making the most of a limited energy budget

In Chapter 27 we talked about 'managing a limited energy budget'. You may find that it helps if, for a while, you keep a note of what you are doing day by day. You may be surprised to find that you are wasting some of your energy on activities that are not that important to you. You may also be able to spot that you are concentrating some activities too close together, when spreading them out during the week would be easier for you.

'Thought' diaries

If you take part in a cognitive behaviour therapy programme for anxiety, panic, depression, or CFS/ME, you may be asked to keep a diary in which you record your thoughts and beliefs. You do not have to be bothered or alarmed by this. Your therapist will give you very clear instructions on how this should be done.

Diary keeping does not have to be a way of life

Some people do find that it helps them to manage themselves better if they make diary keeping a permanent feature of their lives, but it is certainly not essential. On the whole, we have found that keeping specific diaries (such as the ones we have suggested) at definite stages of your self-help programme can be useful, but focusing too much on symptoms can be counterproductive. If you find that you are letting your pacing slip, then it may be helpful to return to keeping an activity diary for a while. If you find yourself in low spirits and think that nothing good ever happens to you, then going back to keeping a satisfaction diary can help to remind you that you do still have good moments. Recording achievements can boost your sense of self-esteem.

You are a unique person and can work out what works for you. As always in this illness, *you* are the person in control and can choose what you do.

However, what we do *not* recommend is keeping the sort of diary that concentrates on 'doom and gloom'. That is likely to lower your spirits in a way that will not do you any good at all.

Appendix 3

Both of these criteria resulted from research scientists getting together to decide definitions of chronic fatigue syndrome that they hoped would improve the process of research into this condition. As we have said before, it is important to be able to compare the results from one research group with those of another, which is not possible if different doctors and scientists are working with different types of patient. We give details of the papers in which these definitions were published in case you want to read the complete reports.

The 'Oxford' definition

Chronic fatigue syndrome (CFS)

- a syndrome characterized by fatigue as the principal symptom

- a syndrome that had a definite onset (not lifelong)
- the symptom of fatigue is severe, disabling, affecting physical and mental functioning, and disproportionate to exertion
- the fatigue should have been present for a minimum of 6 months during which it was present for more than 50 per cent of the time
- other symptoms may be present, particularly myalgia, mood and sleep disturbance.

Exclusions

- Patients with established medical conditions known to produce chronic fatigue (e.g. severe anaemia). Such patients should be excluded whether the medical condition is diagnosed at presentation or only subsequently. All patients should have a history and physical examination performed by a competent physician.
- Patients with a current diagnosis of schizophrenia, manic depressive illness, substance abuse, eating disorder, or proven organic brain disease. Other psychiatric disorders (including depressive illness, anxiety disorders, and hyperventilation syndrome) are not necessarily reasons for exclusion.

Post-infectious fatigue syndrome (PIFS)

There is a subtype of CFS which either follows an infection or is associated with a current infection (although whether such associated infection is of aetiological significance is a topic for research). To meet research criteria for PFIS patients must:

- fulfil the criteria for CFS as defined above, and
- also fulfil the following additional criteria:
  - there is definite evidence of infection at onset or presentation (a patient's self-report is unlikely to be sufficiently reliable)
  - the syndrome is present for a minimum of 6 months after onset of infection
  - the infection has been corroborated by laboratory evidence.

Taken from: Sharpe, M. C., Archard, L. C., Banatvala, J. E., Borysiewicz, L. K., Clare, A. Q., *et al.* (1991). A report—chronic fatigue syndrome: guidelines for research. *Journal of the Royal Society of Medicine*, 84, 118–21.

The International 1994 CDC definition of CFS

Chronic fatigue syndrome (CFS)

Clinically evaluated, unexplained, persistent, or relapsing chronic fatigue of at least 6 months duration which is:

- of new or definite onset (not lifelong)
- not the result of ongoing exertion
- not substantially alleviated by rest, and
- results in substantial reduction in previous levels of occupational, educational, social, or personal activities.

Four or more of the following symptoms are present for a minimum of 6 months:

- impaired memory or concentration
- sore throat

- tender cervical or axillary lymph nodes
- muscle pain (myalgia)
- multijoint pain (arthralgia)
- new type of headaches
- unrefreshing sleep
- postexertional malaise.

Recommended clinical evaluation:

- medical history and physical examination
- mental status evaluation
- laboratory screening by blood and urine tests (a list of such tests is given)
- additional tests as clinically indicated to exclude other diagnoses.

Conditions that exclude a patient from a diagnosis of CFS:

- Any active medical condition that may explain the presence of chronic fatigue
- Any previously diagnosed medical condition whose resolution has not been documented beyond reasonable clinical doubt which may explain the chronic fatiguing illness
- Any past or present diagnosis of serious psychiatric conditions such as:
  - a major depressive disorder with psychotic or melancholic features
  - manic depressive illness
  - schizophrenia
- Eating disorders

- Alcohol or other substance abuse within 2 years of the onset of the chronic fatigue or at any time afterwards
- Severe obesity

Idiopathic chronic fatigue

Clinically evaluated unexplained chronic fatigue that has lasted for a minimum of 6 months but that fails to meet the definition for chronic fatigue syndrome.

Taken from: Fukuda, K., Straus, S. E., Hickie, I., Sharpe, M. C., Dobbins, J. G., Komoroff, A. *et al.* (1994). The chronic fatigue syndrome: a comprehensive approach to its definition and study. *Annals of Internal Medicine*, 121, 953–9.

Appendix 4
Further information

Inevitably, we have not been able to cover everything about CFS/ME in a book of this length. We make some suggestions here of sources of further information.

Research papers

Here is a selection of papers, published in reputable journals, about some of the topics we have discussed throughout the book. We have chosen these to give you more information about research and to demonstrate that what we have said about CFS/ME is backed up by proper research.

Reviews of research and treatment

Levine, P. H. (1998). What we know about chronic fatigue syndrome and its relevance to the practising physician. *American Journal of Medicine*, 105, 1005–35.

Lloyd, A. R., Hickie, I., and Peterson, P. K. (1999). Chronic fatigue syndrome: current concepts of pathogenesis and treatment. *Current Clinical Topics in Infectious Diseases*, 19, 135–59.

Joint Working Party of the Royal Colleges of Physicians, Psychiatrists, and General Practitioners (1996). *Chronic Fatigue Syndrome*. Royal College of Physicians, London.

Reid, S., Chalder, T., Cleare, A. J., Hotopf, M., and Wessely, S. (2000). Chronic fatigue syndrome: clinical review. *British Medical Journal*, 320, 292–6 (a review of Randomized Controlled Trials about the treatment of CFS).

Price, J. R. and Couper, J. (2000). Cognitive behaviour therapy for adults with chronic fatigue syndrome. (Cochrane Review) In *The Cochrane Library*, Issue 1, Oxford Update Software, Oxford.

Research into CBT and GET

Deale, A., Chalder, T., Marks, I., and Wessely, S. (1997). Cognitive behaviour therapy for chronic fatigue syndrome: a randomized controlled trial. *American Journal of Psychiatry*, 154, 408–14.

Sharpe, M., Hawton, K. E., Simpkin, S., Surawy, C., Hackmann, A., Klimes, I. *et al.* (1996). Cognitive behaviour therapy for the chronic fatigue syndrome: a randomized controlled trial. *British Medical Journal*, 312, 22–6.

Sharpe, M. (1998). Cognitive behaviour therapy for chronic fatigue syndrome: efficacy and implications. *American Journal of Medicine*, 105, 104S–9S.

Fulcher, K. Y. and White, P. D. (1997). Randomised controlled trial of graded exercise in patients with the chronic fatigue syndrome. *British Medical Journal*, 314, 1647–52.

Wearden, A. J., Morriss, R. K., Mullis, R., Strickland, P. L., Pearson, D. J. *et al.* (1998). Randomised, double-blind, placebo controlled treatment trial of fluoxetine and graded exercise for chronic fatigue syndrome. *British Journal of Psychiatry*, 172, 485–90.

Help with assessing patient information literature
on treatment choices

Charnock, D., Sheppard, S., Needham, G., and Gann, R.
(1999). DISCERN: an instrument for judging the quality
of written consumer health information on treatment
choices. *Journal of Epidemiology and Community Health*,
53, 105–11. (This gives guidelines both for patients and
for health professionals producing such information. This
information can also be found at the internet address
www.discern.org.uk. We used the DISCERN Instrument
while writing this book.)

Books

We have picked out some books that you might find
helpful if you want to find out more about various
aspects of CFS/ME or about ways in which you can
help yourself. It may seem like a long list, but we are
certainly not suggesting that you should read them all!
Your local library may be able to obtain some of these
for you to borrow.

About CFS/ME

Chronic Fatigue and its Syndromes Simon Wessely,
Matthew Hotopf and Michael Sharpe. Oxford University
Press, 1998—A readable but large textbook, partly
written by one of us. Intended for doctors, this
book takes a comprehensive approach to the whole
question of chronic fatigue as well as CFS/ME. ISBN
0–19–262181–5

**Chronic Fatigue Syndrome: An Integrative Approach to
Evaluation and Treatment** Edited by Mark A. Demitrack
and Susan E. Abbey. The Guildford Press, 1996—

Another textbook for doctors, but easier to read than some. ISBN 1–57230–038–8

Chronic Fatigue Syndrome—Your Questions Answered Dr John Campling and Mrs Frankie Campling. The Erskine Press, 1997—A patient information booklet written largely by one of us and giving a summary of the information in this book. Write to: The Erskine Press, The Old Bakery, Banham, Norwich NR16 2HW enclosing a self addressed 6″ by 9″ envelope and 50 pence. ISBN 1–85297–051–0

A Research Portfolio on Chronic Fatigue Edited by Robin Fox. The Linbury Trust, 1998—An overview of the different areas of research on CFS/ME that have been sponsored by the Linbury Trust. Available free by writing to the Linbury Trust, 9 Red Lion Court, London EC4A 3EB, UK. ISBN 1–85315–367–2

Looking after yourself

The Healing Brain Robert Ornstein and David Sobel. Papermac, 1988—An interesting book about the way that the brain works, focusing on the interactions between the brain and the body. ISBN 0–333–48278–6

Back in Ten Minutes Dr Mary Rintoul and Bernard West. Penguin, 1995—A very practical book about ways to avoid back problems. It contains really clear illustrations of suggested exercises. ISBN 0–14–023482–9

The Which? Guide to Complementary Medicine Barbara Rowlands. Which? Books, 1997—A good guide to complementary and alternative therapies, with sensible suggestions about choosing a therapist. ISBN 0–85202–634–X

Managing More with Less Joanna Howard. Butterworth Heinemann, 1997—Although this book is aimed at people at work, most of what it says can be applied to normal life. ISBN 0–75063–698–X

Help with your emotions

Manage Your Mind Gillian Butler and Tony Hope. Oxford University Press, 1995—One of the best self-help books, covering a wide range of subjects. It is written in a very clear way and is full of common sense. It has good chapters on dealing with worry and anxiety, problem solving, relationships and communication. ISBN 0–19–262383–4

Overcoming Anxiety Helen Kennerley. Robinson, 1998—Self-help techniques for dealing with anxiety. ISBN 1–85487–422–5

Panic Attacks Christine Inghams. Thorsons, 1993—Self-help techniques for dealing with panic. ISBN 0–72252–698–9

Overcoming Depression Paul Gilbert. Robinson, 1997—Self-help techniques for dealing with depression. ISBN 1–85487–434–9

Mind Over Mood Dennis Greenberger and Christine Padesky. Guilford, 1995—One of the best books about cognitive behaviour therapy self-help techniques for dealing with anxiety, panic, and depression. ISBN 0–89862–128–3

Down with Gloom! Professor Brice Pitts. Gaskell, 1993—A brilliant book giving information about what depression is and is not. It is easy to read and has the benefit of funny cartoons by Mel Calman (some of which are very appropriate for CFS/ME). It could be useful if you need to educate those around you about depression. ISBN 0–902241–64–8

Children and young people

Somebody Help ME Jill Moss. Sunbow Books, 1995—A sensible self-help guide for young sufferers. ISBN 0–9525–783–01

A Parent's Guide to CFIDS—How to be an advocate for
your child with Chronic Fatigue Immune Dysfunction
Syndrome David Bell, Mary Robinson, Jean Pollard,
Tom Robinson, and Bonnie Floyd, 1999—An American
guide for parents, particularly looking at education. ISBN
0–20140–797–3

Relaxation

You may decide that you need help in learning how to
relax. Helpful tapes and literature can be obtained by
writing to either:

> Stress Management Institute
> Foxhills, 30 Victoria Avenue
> Shankhill
> Isle of Wight PO37 6LS, UK

or

> Oxford Cognitive Therapy Centre
> Warneford Hospital
> Oxford OX3 7JX, UK

Index

Index

Index